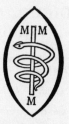

MIND & MEDICINE MONOGRAPHS

Editor

MICHAEL BALINT, M.D., PH.D., M.SC.

19

Contraception and Sexual Life

MIND & MEDICINE MONOGRAPHS
EDITORIAL ADVISORY BOARD

Contraception
and Sexual Life

A THERAPEUTIC APPROACH

L. P. D. TUNNADINE

Foreword by Tom Main

TAVISTOCK PUBLICATIONS

J. B. LIPPINCOTT COMPANY

First published in 1970
by Tavistock Publications Limited
11 New Fetter Lane, London E.C.4
Printed in Great Britain
in 11 point Times New Roman
by Cox & Wyman Ltd, Fakenham, Norfolk

SBN 422 73560 4

Distributed in the United States of America and
in Canada by J. B. Lippincott Company, Philadelphia
and Toronto

Contents

Foreword

BY TOM MAIN

'Not but many useful things might be learnt by that book, but he was laughed at because that art was not to be taught by words, but by practice.'

IZAAK WALTON, *The Compleat Angler*

Dr Tunnadine's book is the result not of scholarship but of thought about clinical skills, experiences, and experiments – the *practices* of herself and her colleagues. She and they discussed their current encounters with patients at Family Planning Clinics, case by case, in weekly seminars with me over the course of a few years. There was no teaching of general principles by me or anybody else, only a dogged study of each clinical encounter, with special emphasis on how the patient dealt with the doctor and how the doctor dealt with the patient. Of course we found each other's work to be full of error, puzzlement, uncertainty, disappointment, strain, and incomprehension in the face of excellent intention, goodwill, patience, and effortful striving. This was inevitable. It is inevitable in every attempt to increase skill, whether it be for fishing, football, carpentry, or doctoring, because practice reveals imperfections that need thought and modification; but only thus can the reward of learning by practice be gained. The acquiring of any skill needs a modification of oneself, a discarding of old habits that have been found useless or even harmful, and the growth, modification, and development of new ones. So it was in this group.

I was the trainer, but I was not the teacher; and could not be, for I was quite unskilled at their work in Family Planning Clinics. On the other hand, I could have taught them, had I wished, how to become more adept at psychiatry or psychoanalysis, for I know something of these disciplines; but this would have been irrelevant for it was not what they sought; they wanted to become better Family Planning Association doctors. In this seminar I was, therefore, another studying colleague, ready, as they were, to try to understand the events they encountered daily. But I had my own viewpoint and background. As a psychoanalyst I was to be aware that things need not always be taken at face value, that there is an unconscious, and that for psychotherapy one needs to listen to, think hard about, and understand patients' communications in depth, and then choose what to convey of one's understanding, and then to observe the effect of that. Then, as a trainer, my orientation had to be less towards supervision of patients than towards the development of doctors. I was also trained in the use of group dynamics, and interested in the use of group processes for training purposes. The methods of the seminar leader in the 'Balint method' of training have, however, already been described *in extenso* by Balint himself,[1] and all I need emphasize here is that in the seminar, of which this book is one fruit, I was not concerned with teaching knowledge but rather with using his method of training for the increase of clinical *skills* in FPA doctors.

The progress of the seminar took classic form. At first the doctors could only use their accustomed medical models for conducting and viewing their work; they reported formally and objectively about patients' complaints, histories and symptoms, and responses to questions; then the results of their examinations and investigations, their own diagnosis of the problems, their treatments and their results. They talked only about patients. It took time for them to review the use-

---

[1] *The Doctor, his Patient and the Illness* by M. Balint. London: Pitman Medical; New York: International Universities Press, 1957.

fulness and limitations of these practices, then to digest the strains of such reviews, and then to grow the courage and freedom even to begin to report about their own contributions towards doctor–patient relation. At first there was dismay as well as relief at the very idea that doctors also have feelings that are decisive for their interventions and that prejudice their attempts at medical objectivity; but we went on to learn at least some of the unthinking habitual patterns of response in each doctor that had interacted with her patients' habitual patterns in ways that were decisive for the outcome of treatment. Lest this seem abrupt, it needs emphasis that it is the merit, as well as the trouble, of discussion with colleagues that others can discern one's patterns more easily than one can oneself; but as all are in the same boat, colleagues, although critical, will also be comradely; and moreover one learns much by observing the skills and errors of colleagues as well as of oneself. So, increasingly, week by week, the doctors reported to each other with less formality and more spontaneity about their weekly work in the new area of interest – the doctor–patient relation. They grew a greater understanding of their patients and themselves, and began to use these understandings to practise in new ways, the results of which could be checked each week. Thus skills grew along with understandings, and non-ritual, thoughtful actions began to replace routine procedures.

With the growth of skills at investigating, understanding, and treating came new findings from among scores of patients, and at last the seminar group began to notice certain *general* principles about the problems of patients. Dr Tunnadine's book is a distillate of these findings and principles.

Our seminar had begun some years later than the pioneer FPA seminar led by Michael Balint, in which I served my apprenticeship and from whom I learned gratefully, but it had its own composition and originality. It did not borrow from the earlier seminar, indeed it could not, but it made its own discoveries – as all seminars should. Many of its findings were not new but with all their merits and demerits, they were original for *it*. Dr Tunnadine's records came from the short-hand notes of the seminar secretary, but the selection of cases and ideas from these to shape a book, the work of compiling it – and the enthusiasm – are entirely her own.

Her book will have much interest for her colleagues in medicine, but its significance does not rest there. It offers pointers towards some of the little-studied fundamentals that lie behind all requests for, or refusals of, contraceptive help in all countries. Now that population control is a problem for mankind, any study that throws any light at all on human sexuality and techniques of investigating it is, literally, vital.

Author's Preface

This book owes its scientific origin to the concept of psycho-physical therapy first developed by Dr Michael Balint in his seminars as long ago as 1958. Among other writers whose work derived from the same source, Leonard J. Friedman, in *Virgin Wives* (1962),[1] applied the technique to the study and treatment of nonconsummation, and Michael Courtenay, in *Sexual Discord in Marriage: a field for brief psychotherapy* (1969),[2] applied it to disharmony in the marital relationship. This book describes its further application to the emotional problems of contraceptive gynaecology, and to the wider field of female sexual anxiety and frigidity.

The fact that the technique has been developed to apply to such a wide area of human distress is tribute to the thinking of Dr Balint and his early colleagues. That the present group, which began wholly independently in 1960, on its own programme of learning and discovery, has found the technique successful in these wider applications, is surely ample confirmation, if such were needed, of its truly scientific validity.

A group of doctors working for the Family Planning Association began in 1960 to meet under the leadership of Dr Tom Main, a psychoanalyst with special interest in group training methods, to study the marital problems of the

[1] Mind and Medicine Monograph No. 5, London: Tavistock; Philadelphia and Toronto: Lippincott.
[2] Mind and Medicine Monograph No. 16, London: Tavistock; Philadelphia and Toronto: Lippincott.

patients they saw in their normal clinic work, and to learn and develop methods of helping them. In the course of this study we came to understand something of the nature of sexual anxiety in the female, and of frigidity itself. We found that, just as sexual intercourse is both a physical and an emotional affair, so are its problems neither purely physical nor purely emotional, but rather the result of a woman's emotional attitudes upon her physical performance. It is not surprising, therefore, that by learning how to apply the principles and insights of the psychotherapeutic approach to the physical and gynaecological transactions that occur in a contraceptive clinic, we achieved more fruitful results than may be available either in purely physical gynaecology, or in purely psychological therapy or emotional counselling.[1]

The gynaecologist who is trained to discuss his patients' feelings is rare, although there is no reason why he or the family doctor should not learn to do so. The marriage counsellor, priest-confessor, or psychoanalyst who examines his patients' genitals is nonexistent, and for him to do so would clearly be inappropriate. It became clear that the FPA clinic worker had other special advantages in this field. Various factors contributed to this. The doctors were mostly married women, and worked in a setting – the birth-control clinic – in which it is implicit in the very nature of the service that sexual matters are proper subjects for discussion. One may go further, and suggest that it is also implicit that intercourse is not only for conceiving babies, but for the expression of a relationship – for pleasure – if contraceptive advice is offered in conscience at all.

I am often asked why FPA doctors should concern themselves with the psyche. Are there not already enough 'enthusiastic amateurs' seeking to dabble in people's sexual lives? The answer is clear. Just as the Family Planning Movement itself arose in direct response to the needs of the patients, so this work became necessary because a fast-increasing

[1] Cf. Friedman, *Virgin Wives* (1962).

number of our patients sought such help – and because we found the existing methods of treatment were not good enough.

The birth-control clinic is today a very different thing in different parts of the world. In Asia, for example, where population control is an urgent contribution to freedom from hunger, the need is for expediency, economy, and comprehensibility. Doctors working in such areas may well feel that subtleties of preference have to wait. It was the late Pandit Nehru who said one needed a full belly before one worried about democracy. Even so, it may be necessary to study emotional attitudes in order to understand the problems of acceptability and motivation. Similarly, in many places that would feel insulted by the term 'underdeveloped', women still grow ill and die from conceiving more pregnancies than they are fit to bear. Here family planning is still preventive medicine in the physical sense.

It has been increasingly true, however, in the last twenty years, that most of our patients are a far cry from the downtrodden wives for whom this work in England was pioneered. We meet healthy young women with mortgages and washing machines, apparently seeking only to plan their families in a rational manner. I say apparently because, although the FPA is a vast and fast-expanding independent health service, seeing tens of thousands of patients annually, birth control still means for the majority in this country, either the pill from the family doctor, or the sheath from the slot-machine. Those who do come to FPA clinics are thus to that extent a self-selected group.

We find among such patients thousands who, given the atmosphere in which intimate confidences are possible, will express the wish for help with the quality of their sexual lives. Some years ago a group of senior FPA doctors recognized this. They recognized too that the advice they were giving – the books they were lending – was not enough if the problem was more than superficial. I emphasize that these were experienced women, not only in sexual gynaecology, but with families and sexual lives of their own.

Thus this work began. These doctors began to meet with Dr Balint to try to do better. Because of the scientific excitement and clinical success engendered by their studies, the present group was set up soon after with Dr Main. Although we owed to the pioneers the original concept of psychophysical therapy, we were in every sense a new group, with a new leader, who allowed us no preconceptions. Indeed, by the time *Virgin Wives* was published, it was already clear that such a group cannot merely be a learning group, but is by definition a discovery group. We worked case by case, doctor by doctor, examining our own techniques and prejudices as well as the patients' problems. Thus we came to find some of the concepts explored in *Virgin Wives* confirmed and elaborated by a different route, and other concepts altogether fresh emerging.

What was certain was that this technique works, and bears the test of science in that it can be taught to other wholly independent workers who will then find the results reproduced.

The cases quoted here are factual. No patient need fear, however, that professional secrecy has been betrayed. The material described is a distillate of work studied by thirteen doctors over five years. The total caseload from which it was selected for inclusion is estimated at over 20,000 patients.

This book is not intended as a training manual, but as an introductory outline of the understanding that seminar training alone can, we believe, provide. To those doctors for whom it stimulates interest in training we can confidently forecast a new dimension in clinical experience. To those potential patients and other interested parties who may read it, we hope to indicate that another form of help is at hand. This FPA training scheme is expanding rapidly, and has by now embraced some 200 doctors, a number of whom have qualified to train others. It is hoped that this skill may soon be available to patients in every branch.

The scheme has been financed by the Lord and Lady Monckton Fund. Through it, Nancy Raphael and a handful of her supporters have managed to keep the training scheme going within the FPA, which we hope may go from strength to strength. To them, therefore, we, and I believe this branch of medicine, owe deep thanks for their vision, courage, and generosity.

I wish to thank also my secretary, Gillian Wood, who found time to type and correct the manuscript despite two full-time jobs and the expectation of a third; Dr Tom Main for his foreword, setting this work into its context from the psychological point of view; and Rosemarie Lincoln and Mary Yirrell for correcting the proofs.

My personal thanks are due above all to my colleagues in the original 'Monday Group', who contributed not only to the substance of this book, but to my education also. Alexandra Tobert in particular spent many hours with me on the original material. They were; Dr Nest Crane, Dr Rosemary Heaf, Dr Geraldine Howard, Dr Olive Hurford, Dr Barbara Law, Dr Rosemarie Lincoln, Dr Ann Reader, Dr Robina Thexton, Dr Alexandra Tobert; and in the beginning Dr Michael Courtenay, Dr Elsie Shinberg, and Dr Joy West.

I dedicate the book to them, and to Dr Tom Main, who led us, and without whom we could have achieved nothing. He will deem this a doubtful compliment, since he believes this therapeutic technique is taught and learned only by the living dynamics of clinical experience within the seminar system, and not, repeat not, from books of this kind.

He is, of course, absolutely right.

CHAPTER 1

The Interview

It is hoped the reader will gather that the technique consists not so much of following a list of instructions, as of conducting a consultation in a particular manner. In this sense it has much in common with the seminar method by which we learned it. We proceed with the patient, not by teaching her facts, or by giving her advice from our own experience, but by appreciating her own attitudes and showing them to her in such a way that she comes to see them for herself. Similarly, the seminar doctors were not taught formal theories of one psychological school or another. Instead, their method of handling each patient was examined by the group in such a way that they came to see for themselves how their prejudices and faulty techniques hampered them in treating each patient.

It became clear at an early stage that each doctor contributed, by her very personality, a blanket approach to her patients, which differed from that of other doctors. This was in each case not necessarily good or bad – only indiscriminate. It took no account of the fact that patients too differ. A fine approach to one patient might be useless to the next. For example, there were 'teaching doctors' who would offer anatomy or physiology lessons, most helpful to a patient whose only problem was her ignorance. But these patients proved to be rare – we are on the whole a literate society –

and such lessons were little use to, for example, the physio-therapist, whose knowledge was of honours degree standard, but whose emotional reaction was that the vagina was an organ of clinical biology, about which tender feelings and anxieties were inappropriate.

Other doctors, like other patients, had an 'athletic' approach to the sexual act. They would advise pillows placed here, or muscles moved there, as though with enough training and practice the Gold Medal would be theirs. Fine for the patient needing such encouragement, and practical and un-inhibited enough in temperament to use it. Not so, however, for the patient whose upbringing made her feel it wicked even to wish to enjoy sex, never mind wilfully to experiment and practice. Not so either for the girl whose problem was the lack of romance and sentiment in her husband's already highly commendable athletic efforts.

Other doctors were warmly encouraging – 'Come on in,' we implied, 'The water's fine – sex is lovely (*I* think!).' Such an attitude from an apparently respectable woman was often very useful for the girl whose own mother had seemed shy or prohibitive. But for the girl who felt her own sexual desires to be disgusting, the reaction was shocked disapproval. Small wonder that such patients sometimes did not return to such sexy-seeming doctors.

All this we came to see, case by case, until each doctor began, painfully, to recognize her blind spots. Then at last she could begin to 'aim off', allowing for this, and recognize the effect she was having on different patients. Now the difference between patients became clear, the doctor's prejudices could recede, and the patient's own contribution come under objective scrutiny.

We learned first to listen rather than to question and talk – and to be in every sense 'aware'. One observes not only the words spoken by each patient but her appearance and manner, and tries to understand. One not only observes the outward features, mode of dress and grooming, but asks

2

oneself what these may signify in terms of the problem at hand. A patient who adopts a style younger than her years, like 'mutton dressed as lamb', may not do so by accident. She may have difficulty in accepting maturity. Heavy make-up may be a matter of high fashion. It may equally suggest a patient's need to disguise something in herself. A sophisticated or business-like demeanour may reveal anxieties about showing weakness or dependency. A patient who knows it all may be one who has difficulty in admitting her need for help.

There is another level at which these observations must be noted and understood before any useful action can be taken. This is in terms of the 'doctor–patient relationship'. In the short-term, brief-encounter therapy, which is all the clinic doctor has at her disposal for purely practical reasons – and this is surely even more true for the busy family doctor – this acquired consciousness of the effect different patients have on our own feelings is one of the most vital tools of our trade. We use it, and the 'moment of truth', to which I shall refer presently, as short cuts to our understanding of the patient, as another therapist might use drugs or hypnosis.

Briefly it may be said that a doctor's feelings vary from patient to patient, and that this is not an accident. The patient contributes to it, and her contribution is often a reflection of her effect upon other people in her life.

For example, the doctor may find herself liking a patient and sympathizing and identifying with her. This is very pleasant, and perhaps in general medicine very useful. In this work it must be noted. It may mean the patient can admit no fault in herself, cannot allow aggressive feelings to come to the surface, or simply cannot tolerate unpleasantness. 'I felt she reacted just as I would have done,' reported one doctor of a patient who had incidentally laid the blame firmly upon her husband and had elicited from the doctor a letter referring him, whom she had never seen, for treatment! It was not hard to imagine the husband's difficulty with such a wife. Whatever

3

was wrong, it surely could not be her fault. What a burden is perfection in others – no wonder his erections were failing.

The patient who continually asks questions or insists her problem is purely physical may be right. On the other hand, it may prove that she dare not examine her deeper feelings or allow them to be explored because she feels they are too terrible to share, or even admit to herself. Such women have often submitted to – no, insisted upon is more accurate – repeated surgery rather than face the idea that their feelings might be at fault.

The patient who sits passively, forcing the doctor to ask questions or offer suggestions, may also not do so by accident. She may be one who cannot contribute herself but must be bullied into things by other people. Such patients are often the same in intercourse, and their husbands find themselves trying everything short of standing on their heads, without evoking any response.

Another similar facet is the obedience of some patients. They come to the clinic on time, make no fuss, and do all they are told by doctor or parent. Model patients, one might think, and model daughters. All that is missing is any contribution from themselves. This may be very aggressive behaviour indeed, causing impotence in doctor and husband alike. It is that effective fighting force we call 'passive resistance' or 'dumb insolence'. Such patients need to be put in touch with the resentments within themselves before they can loosen up sufficiently for examination of their underlying fears.

In the time and atmosphere which the normal clinic consultation imposes upon us, we concentrate therefore upon two facets of observable fact – not hearsay – which are revealed to us by conscious awareness of our own feelings. While other therapists concern themselves with the patient's circumstances and history, we concern ourselves with the patient's reaction to them, as expressed to us in the here-and-now. While others concentrate upon the patient's reactions upon others in their lives, we concentrate upon their effect on us in the here-and-now. The understanding of these reactions is to some extent a matter of experience, and we have not learned it by reading textbooks of psychology. The seminar method of training has shown it to us in the way in which our reporting of cases reveals the feeling between doctor and patient. Every doctor can feel. If the feelings which each patient provokes can be noted, understanding requires only the awareness of one basic fact of human behaviour. This is that every attitude has its reverse side. We do not show emotion, or conceal it, in a vacuum. A person who hides all feeling must have feeling to hide, and the stronger her need to hide it, the stronger may that feeling be. A calmly accepted emotion does not require protestations of denial. A woman who denies all interest in sex must feel there is something undesirable in being interested, while a patient who appears very 'hot stuff' may be trying to hide her sexual inadequacies. In handling the doctor, the patient provokes feelings in the doctor as she provokes them in others. This is the sort of person she is. If the doctor finds herself bullying or cajoling, then the patient needs to be bullied or cajoled. Why? If the doctor is involved in a fight, then the patient has picked one. Why? If the consultation is all sweetness and light, then the patient needs it so. Why? And if the patient reveals no feeling, she needs to hide it. Why?

We have touched upon how the patient's treatment of the doctor may reflect her treatment of her husband. It is important to stress also how often the doctors in the group have found themselves placed by their patients in the maternal role. Again, not all patients do this. Some are so independent as to be unable to concede the need for our help as doctors, never mind as mothers. Nor were the actual comparative ages of patient and doctor relevant here. Few of the doctors were of an age to have adult children, and many patients who acted the child's role were over twenty-five. The observation that one was in a mother–child relationship was itself often of diagnostic value, in that here was a patient who was still

5

emotionally more daughter than lover or wife. We could often proceed further to observe and interpret what manner of daughter this was – obedient, rebellious, or seeking attention, love, or punishment. We found too that in terms of treatment this realization between doctor and patient could be of positive therapeutic value, particularly when maternal prohibition or 'non-permission' was at the root of a woman's sexual anxiety.

One might expect in the still largely one-sex atmosphere of the FPA clinic, occasionally though regrettably frankly feminist, that many doctor–patient relationships would have Lesbian undertones. This possibility was examined by the group when relevant, and was found to be surprisingly rare. Clearly, when the doctor felt such tensions, she received in them clues to the patient's anxiety or marital difficulty. On the whole, however, the mother–child one-sex relationship was much more common. More common still was the relationship of two adult women in the sex business, sharing the tacit understanding that the doctor wished for the patient what she wished for herself – a rich and fulfilling sexual life.

In trying to analyse the significance of the doctor–patient relationship the accent has been on understanding. This indeed is half the battle, just as in all medicine diagnosis is half the treatment. We are far, however, from the early concept of the psychotherapist as a passive mirror for a patient's attitudes. The doctor's positive contribution is more difficult to analyse, because it consists in every case and at every moment of 'playing by ear'. Each doctor will employ her instinct and experience to decide when to interpret her understanding, when to encourage, when to attack, when to be permissive, when to hold her peace and allow the patient to run on until her exaggerated reactions thus become obvious even to herself. But act, advise, and encourage we do, as well as using the classic interpretative technique. Here our work differs from that of the true psychotherapist. But the unique

6

quality of this work lies chiefly in the use we make of the physical clinic transactions – vaginal examination, cap-fitting, cap-teaching, etc. The application of psychological insight to these matters has helped our understanding and the patient's recovery with such consistency that we have come to speak of the 'moment of truth'.

CHAPTER 2

The Moment of Truth

We find the moment of vaginal examination to be a moment of great importance to our patients. As will be shown repeatedly throughout the text, it seems to provide a kind of entrée to genuine feeling, as though layers of inhibition are shed with the clothes, and the baring of the genital area carries with it a baring of the patient's feelings about it. It is, of course, a moment of some desperation for the patient, as though all that has been kept hidden from the outside world, by carefully built defences – modesty, civilized and moral attitudes and behaviour – is now about to be shared with another person: the doctor. While we examine dozens of patients each week of our lives, so that embarrassment or distaste has been long abandoned, to the patient herself what is to be revealed may be something most intimate and secret. It may also be, to her, nasty or dirty or prohibited or feared, or unlike other people's and therefore abnormal. It may on the other hand be unbearably exciting or wonderful – so exciting or wonderful as to be frightening or shameful. She may think it too small, so that intercourse will 'tear her apart' or 'be like smashing through a brick wall'. Some have feared it led to a great cavern the size of a full-term uterus, or to the rectum or abdominal cavity, so that things might be lost in or damaged by it. Others thought that there was only one passage, through which all 'dirty' things came. Others feel it to be so prohibited and secret as to be impossible to speculate about at all; they may then deny themselves all knowledge, and harbour strange fantasies despite a perfectly sound theoretical awareness of its true nature.

At a more superficial level of consciousness, a patient may fear that vaginal examination will reveal to the doctor facts she does not wish to acknowledge – that she is, or is not, a virgin; that she has some abnormality, real or imagined, which she attributes to masturbation, or illegal abortion, or venereal disease. To the doctor who meets them every day, and is in any case not sitting in moral judgement, these fears may seem foolish and unimportant. To the patient they are very meaningful, and may make the thought of examination a matter of great strain and fear. It is thus in using these moments, and through the business of teaching the patient to examine herself and to fit her cap, which often follows in normal clinic procedure, that the specifically psychophysical aspect of our method is found to be most relevant and most useful.

At first we chose the moment to examine our patients physically almost at random. We then came to notice how sometimes we would do it when our exploration of the patient's feelings came to an uncomfortable pause. We came to see that we were thus using examination as an escape from the discomfort of a 'heavy-going' or a too emotionally disturbing situation. A sullen, unresponsive, argumentative or weeping patient put us on the defensive. We therefore retreated to the safe ground of being clever physical doctors, taking command of the situation by physical examination. Once this was understood, we tried instead to understand how the patient made us do this, and to show her instead why it happened.

Having explored the patient's fantasies as far as possible, however, and decided rationally that the moment for examination is appropriate, we watch carefully the patient's

9

reaction to it. Some ask frankly what to do – that is, they need to be told. Others reveal unusual modesty in their shedding of immaculate undies, or apologize for not having bathed. Others still, now that all is to be revealed, produce for the first time their real fear – that there is cancer, or 'something nasty' or unnatural, inside. The patient's attitude on the couch itself will also be revealing. She may be very businesslike or passive, showing her difficulty in revealing feelings of fear or uncertainty. Or she may show in her physical resistance to examination what physical difficulties she presents to her husband in intercourse. A patient who has asked for surgical investigations or practical advice about subfertility without any hint of difficulty in intercourse, may reveal clearly at this time that intercourse has never taken place – not only because her hymen is intact but because she will shoot up off the couch with knees pressed tight together at the very approach of the examining finger. It is vital, then, to be aware and sensitive, and not to rush on with exhortations and reassurance which will make her fears seem foolish or painful. She knows they are foolish and painful. This is why she has come.

At first it was the positive revelations of fear or distaste or resistance we noted most fully. Later we came to pay equal attention and tribute to negative 'moments of truth'. The patient who tries hard – obviously hard – to be sensible or practical or impassive at this moment is showing us something of her defence system – something of her difficulties in intercourse. Abandonment to the depths and heights of sexual love is not compatible with good sense and practicality and modest 'Sunday-best behaviour'. The 'relaxation' so vaunted in our manuals and homilies must be emotional relaxation. Physical relaxation alone is, after all, one step short of going to sleep.

We may learn, then, something of the patient's problem in intercourse, and something too of her fantasies about the nature of her own genital apparatus. Having shared, explored, and perhaps interpreted something of these feelings, we may

10

proceed to confront her with the reality of the matter. It is usual, when a diaphragm is to be the birth-control method, to teach the patient to fit it herself, and to feel inside the vagina to check its position. She is encouraged to feel the rim of the cap sitting behind and above the bony symphysis pubis, and then to feel on up to the cervix and to recognize it, so that she may assure herself that it is covered by the cap. Many patients express feelings of surprise or anxiety or distaste at this moment. 'It is not as small as I thought', 'Can I damage myself?', 'I thought there should be a wall across – does it mean I am not a virgin?', 'It feels horrible – like an open wound', or merely, 'I couldn't possibly let anything inside'. All these responses may be heard, explored, and interpreted. If the patient has had a chance to recognize her feelings about her inside, the realization of the true facts is often a great and curative relief to her. It has been enough to cure nonconsummation, and a healthy husband's resulting impotence, overnight. The contrast with fact and fantasy seems curative only when the fantasy has been adequately explored. Without this, books, diagrams, lectures, are rarely effective.

There is another mechanism by which this teaching of examining the vagina produces remarkable therapeutic results. This is with the girl who has taken into herself prohibitions on sexuality, and on touching herself, from her mother. Whatever the mother's actual attitude may have been, to these girls 'She never told me' means 'She thought I should not know. Ergo, it is bad'. The vagina is a hidden and therefore secret and mysterious part of the body, unlike the penis, whose purpose and sensation are obvious from an early age. To this may be added the 'Don't touch' idea, often associated with the patient's feeling of the wickedness of masturbatory pleasure. The unwarned and unheralded onset of menstruation may also add to the 'not nice' concept of the vagina, particularly when the only information has come, not from an understanding mother, but from the salacious reports of giggling schoolfellows. In any event, the handing-over of this organ and permission to enjoy it, by a respectable mother-figure, the doctor, who has already shared her anxieties, again seems to operate as a confrontation of fantasy with fact. The fantasy: this part is bad, prohibited, still belonging to mother who has not handed over permission for a sexual life. The fact: a motherly woman says, 'Go ahead – it is yours to explore, use, love with, just like your lips or hands: a decent beautiful organ of pleasure.'

CHAPTER 3

Factual Teaching and Reassurance

It is interesting that we have found these well-tried assets of normal medical advice useless when the problem is more than superficial. Reassurance we have indeed often found to be worse than useless, since it may let the patient and doctor off the emotional hook at moments of high feeling. To soothe a patient who needs to let rip with her fears or resentments is tantamount to saying, 'That is enough. Pull yourself together. I can't stand this painful emotion either.' The temptation to do so may be strong. We have met situations where, even though the doctor may try to keep her head, a patient's disturbing show of deep emotion has provoked a nurse or trainee, for example, to move so far from her professional role as to intervene with offers of books to read or exhortations to 'pull yourself together'. She cannot stand the tension and defends herself unconsciously by telling the patient in effect to 'shut up'. This is, of course, a therapeutic disservice, reinforcing rather than relieving the patient's own distress at the 'exhibition' she feels she is making.

The question of factual instruction is also interesting from the technical viewpoint. We find that without the exploration of fantasy and anxiety we have described, factual teaching, however warmly and encouragingly done, can only be accepted and taken in by individual patients according to their own emotional capacity. This may be of interest to those who must decide how and when to instruct their young. The fear is that too much knowledge too soon encourages them to go forth and experiment. To illustrate that for many this is not so, we cite a group of patients who were all professional women with ample factual knowledge who nevertheless were emotionally unable to use their knowledge.

A physiotherapist had nearly finished her training, so however incomplete childhood instruction had been, her knowledge of human anatomy and physiology was by now extensive. She came before marriage, ostensibly for a cap. Not until she was about to be examined did she reveal any anxiety. She then confessed to fear of pain in intercourse, and showed complete ignorance of her sexual anatomy. The doctor, not then specially trained, was unable to interpret her denial of knowledge, and fitted her with a cap and taught her to stretch herself in the usual way. The patient complained of acute nausea at this, and nearly fainted. A week later she returned, supported by her fiancé and said she had never really wanted a cap – they would use sheaths. Here was a patient who, the doctor now realizes, was screaming by her behaviour, 'This is not a cap problem. I am afraid, and need help to come to terms with sexuality. I am so anxious that I cannot even admit to myself that I know what it is like – never mind touch it or use it for intercourse.'

A girl who complained of 'lack of libido' was a highly intelligent schoolteacher who kept the doctor in her place by quoting textbooks of psychology and 'knowing all about sex', yet was completely frigid after two years of marriage. In this case her protestations of superior knowledge were part of her problem. She had to be 'on top' of her class at school, of the doctor in the interview, and of her husband by keeping control of the intercourse situation. Her intellect, so far from helping her to be a good lover, was her defence against the foolish dependency she feared should she let herself go in the submission of an orgasm.

Another patient insisted on equality with the doctor by brandishing books and insisting she knew all about the facts of conception. She even volunteered a temperature chart with ovulation peaks nicely demonstrated. Yet she complained of subfertility, knowing that she allowed intercourse only when conception was impossible. Her problem was not what it seemed, but her anxiety about her sexual wishes, which she denied by saying cultural interests were more important. She too had to be put in touch with her less competent side – her wish to be earthy and dependent – the femininity that was too exciting to admit.

A research biologist who knew in minute detail all about her body emphasized her one-upmanship with the doctor by stressing this scientific knowledge. She could, however, allow intercourse only about once a month, and then found it difficult to achieve at all. Her husband had thus been rendered incapable of emission, and his erections too were beginning to flag. Such is the power of a controlling woman, as we shall see repeatedly in the cases that follow. It seems this girl too was so fearful of being weak or dependent that she had to control not only herself but all about her with efficiency and cleverness.

Our final example of this pattern was an experienced nursing sister who also made it difficult for the doctor to be a doctor by her 'I know as much about it as you' attitude. At the moment of examination this woman remarked, 'I know all about relaxation. I have been doing exercises for years.' She was, however, completely frigid until put in

15

touch with the babyish side of herself which longed to reverse roles and be taken care of by others. It is important to understand and to show such patients that it is something in themselves they are needing to control, and that they reveal this in the way they control others.

CHAPTER 4

The Language of Symbolism

It has been stressed that the doctors in our seminar have not had a formal course of lectures in the conventional sense, and that we have not sought to become trained psychoanalysts. We are not, therefore, deeply steeped in Freudian symbolism. One of our leader's maxims when we tended to become fanciful was 'An aeroplane is a phallic symbol. It is also a very useful means of transport!' Nevertheless, certain aspects of this language have come into our experience with such clarity and consistency that they have become tools of our trade. We recognize their significance and can interpret them usefully to our patients.

Certain masculine symbols occur from time to time. We noted the resentment of one patient who felt her husband's orgasm was more exciting than her own, and who said she wished he spent more time on her and less on his car. Another used a similar symbol in saying that, as a child, she had thought boys' toys more interesting than girls'. Recognition of this symbolism makes it easy to interpret to such a patient that the penis seems better than the vagina, and to explore her feelings that a woman is an inferior thing to be. Obviously she cannot expect wonderful things from what she sees as a poor piece of apparatus, and she must be helped to value her vagina as a good organ of feeling and expression in its own right.

Since most of our patients are women, and we are dealing with feelings about their genital apparatus and sexual performance, most of the symbolism we encounter is related to these. We have in illustration a rich vocabulary about houses, (vaginae), furnishings, housework, and the like. This equation of 'house' with vagina is absolutely justified in our experience.

One patient was angry with her mother who, she felt, had not given her permission to own her vagina. 'The trouble is,' she said, 'that we live in my mother's house. She does my washing and cooks my meals.' The reference to preparation of meals is also often met in terms of the responsibility for love-making. 'I go to a lot of trouble to get it nice for him. Then he wolfs it down and leaves me to clear up the mess.' A gift to a doctor with the sensitivity to reply, 'It sounds rather like the way you feel about intercourse.' Some patients report putting their cap, or accepting the penis, into their vagina on the same day as they take possession of their new house. Another said she would like to give up her job and spend more time on the house, doing silly feminine things. This reflected perfectly her dilemma between her sensible competent defence system and her wishes to be a feminine dependent 'housewife' – which the career-girl in her saw as 'silly'.

A girl who lived in her mother's house came for pre-marital cap-fitting, saying that she and her husband did not want a baby until they had a house of their own. This is not unreasonable in practical terms, and a common enough remark. In this case, however, it symbolized neatly the pattern of anxiety she subsequently revealed. She was still emotionally tied to her mother, regardless of the housing situation, and was unable to enjoy intercourse while her mother was not only inside the house but, as it were, inside her own head. This patient demanded practical hints from the doctor, and was angry when she did not get them – a reflection of resentment towards her mother for not telling her anything. A truer interpretation was, 'I could not allow myself to hear anything from my mother.' Therefore the doctor was able to suggest to her that she could not allow *herself* to have sexual wishes or to take an active part in sex. The mother, the doctor, the husband, had to do all the work and take all the responsibility. Shown this, she began to improve, and at the moment of vaginal examination was able to confess that what spoiled intercourse for her was that she longed to hold her husband eagerly to her, but something (her internal prohibitions blamed on her mother) held her back and broke the spell. Her mounting feeling of prohibited excitement was thus switched off.

CHAPTER 5

The Unspoken Communication

It is rare for a woman to walk into an FPA clinic and say, 'I do not enjoy intercourse. Please help me.' This may sometimes be because she feels it is expected of her to ask for contraceptive advice. We must also remember, however, that where frigidity or other sexual anxiety exists it is often of the nature of the problem that the woman has difficulty in admitting that she does not enjoy intercourse because she has internal doubts about its being a proper thing to desire. Likewise a frigid woman is often one who has internal difficulties in asking for help at all.

We have to learn, therefore, to be alert to ways in which women may reveal their anxieties without being able to express them verbally. Such 'communications by behaviour' occur constantly in our experience, and indicate the need for further exploration. Coming to the clinic in itself conveys something about the patient. These implications are important to understand, not only for doctors, but also for those who decide clinic policies.[1] We know that, for many patients who come apparently foolishly or cynically, the problem is not what it seems. If they are turned away because we see only

[1] See J. Pasmore and M. Blair, Family Planning for the Unmarried, *Journal of The Royal College of General Practitioners,* vol. 18, p. 214, October, 1969.

20

their apparent irrationality or 'immorality', the opportunity to help them to improve their sexual lives is lost. It may often be months or years before they find the courage to try again, since their fear that their needs are foolish and improper will have been harshly confirmed.

Premarital Patients

Not long ago, many FPA clinics demanded documented evidence of a marriage date less than six weeks ahead before an unmarried girl was admitted. Today, most clinics admit even those with no marriage plans, but much heart-searching about the propriety of this still occurs among doctors as well as lay people. Our now wide experience confirms absolutely the necessity of seeing each individual as a patient – a person with feelings and possibly with difficulties – rather than as a social problem or a licence-seeking sinner.

While many patients seek contraceptive advice alone, and reveal no underlying emotional problem even to the trained observer, certain facets of the attendance of others are pointers to the possibility of such problems.

Some patients come long before marriage is planned, having arranged a long engagement. One such came 'just to inquire' nine months before the appointed day; sent away with books and advice to return three months before the wedding, she soon returned complaining of a discharge – a symptom we have often noticed may indicate the feeling of 'something nasty' inside. Examination was impossible, and fear of intercourse was subsequently revealed, discussed, and removed. Her fantasy was that it would be 'awful', both in the damaging and the wicked sense. After two interviews cap-fitting was possible and the wedding-date was advanced.

To many it is clear that the engagement brings to the surface panic fears that have been pushed to the background of consciousness until the realization that on a given day this terrifying thing – intercourse – will happen. Any premarital

21

patient, therefore, who is difficult to examine, or who finds cap-fitting difficult, or who is obviously gritting her teeth or needing to pluck up courage, may be thus revealing fears she is unable to verbalize. Many if inadequately treated come back, if they dare, complaining of nonconsummation or frigidity.

This anxiety pattern is not confined to those with engage-ment rings. We meet many who, apparently 'living in sin', have similarly been unable to consummate their affairs; and others who, brazenly it seems, asking for birth-control advice 'just in case', can use the opportunity, if offered, to reveal terror or revulsion about the prospect of intercourse.

Conversely, many who seem frankly promiscuous have never enjoyed intercourse. Our clinical experience makes non-sense of the idea that they are merely lustful pleasure-seekers whose untrammelled sexual appetites need only the curb of discipline. Many greet the question 'Do you enjoy it to the full?' or 'Is it all you hoped for?' from a respectable doctor who seems concerned that they should, with astonishment. Our very acceptance that they may have needs of this kind is enough to allow all kinds of fears, fantasies, and pain to be revealed.

A nineteen-year-old, totally masked as a person by her long dirty hair, massive eye-shadow, leather jacket, and grubby jeans, was less than endearing in her 'want to make something of it?' demeanour. She said she supposed she had better go on the pill, since she had already had one baby at fifteen and an abortion just recently 'from an old girl around the corner'. Although everyone said she had better stop it, the only kicks she had were thumbing rides on lorries. Her home town was a 'one-eyed hole'. This attitude persisted despite the doctor's interpretation that she seemed to want to shock her, although the patient for the first time blinked at this and looked her straight in the eye in sur-prise. At examination she sighed theatrically, 'Oh, this drag again.' When the doctor interpreted, 'It doesn't sound as though you find this part of you very romantic or beautiful', the 'brazen hussy' crumpled in a flash into a weeping child. Intercourse had been 'nothing'. At home 'they were only happy if she was out of the way'. Her fruitless quest from stranger to stranger was for the love and tenderness – 'the real thing' – which she had never known at home.

The doctor's response was not that intercourse was something to be stopped – she needed to relate deeply to another person – but something she needed help to do well. One more interview based on the parallel between her need for help from the doctor and her need to get close to her parents, was enough to allow her to return home, get a steady job helping in their shop, and begin to discuss her needs with her mother. Another few months, during which she learned to put in a cap without distaste, but in fact never used it in action, and she could say that her vagina was 'not such a mess as she thought'. She wrote to the doctor not long afterwards saying that she had met a 'smashing fellow' – all the men before had been faceless ciphers – that intercourse was wonderful, and that they were saving to get married.

Other patients may reveal an anxiety they cannot verbalize by causing a stir in the clinic; by feeling faint or nauseated at examination or cap-fitting; or by always contriving to be the first or the last in the queue. Here too the 'aware' doctor may find time to show the patient that she can recognize worry when she sees it, and may thus enable the patient to elaborate or to complain. Many deep but treatable anxieties have been detected in just this way.

The Irrational Visit

The irrational visit must be seen for what it may be, an unspoken communication of the need to air an 'unspeakable' problem. People can, of course, be just stupid, but they are not usually wilfully so. Like the patient who came, apparently far too soon, for her premarital advice, others come when such advice is clearly unnecessary. Some are obviously pregnant already, but their request for a general discussion may well mask fears about confinement itself, or about their capacity for motherhood.

Another patient, grey-haired and obviously post-menopausal, wandered in 'thinking this was the smear clinic', although large notices proclaimed that this was not so. A sensitive lay-worker suggested she might like a word with the doctor anyway, now she was here. Examination revealed her to be virgo intacta, and she was able to admit her longing for a sexual life 'but I suppose it is too late, doctor'. Despite a certain degree of vaginal atrophy, this psycho-physical technique did result after two visits in a degree of consummation and sexual pleasure that was tremendously rewarding for this couple in their late fifties. Resentments of her husband for being 'too gentle' were aired and forgotten. She learned to stretch and lubricate the introitus and found it much easier than she dreamed – she had always thought it had to be 'broken in'. So age and the passage of time, which so often make the doctor share the patient's hopeless despair, are not of themselves a barrier to useful therapy.

The Last-minute Communication

This patient illustrates also a phenomenon most important in the understanding of clinic behaviour, which we call the last-minute communication. Like her, many women who have not previously found the courage to seek help with unsatisfactory sexual lives, find that the approach of the menopause, or perhaps the marriage of a daughter, brings to the surface a desperation to become a woman, as it were, before it is too late. They therefore come for a smear or for contraceptive advice, or on some other respectable pretext. The doctor who recognizes and elicits from them a story of frigidity often feels despair and panic that it is indeed too late to help. This is a reflection of such feelings in the patient. Sharing this interpretation with the patient is in itself an encouragement to someone whose problem is, at least in part, that she doubts the legitimacy of her wishes.

Similarly, the premarital patient who comes only a few days before the wedding, or the night before she is due to fly to another country, so that useful advice seems impossible, may be thus revealing the difficulties she has had in daring to come at all. The doctor who, infected by her panic, sends her away with a packet of sheaths and instructions to come back when there is more time may reinforce her fears that anxiety is foolish, that her first intercourse is something to be 'got over' with a stiff upper-lip, and so on. To pay tribute to the obvious panic situation and allow the anxiety to be aired takes only a few moments and ensures that the patient will find it easier to return.

Finally, every experienced family doctor will confirm our finding that the true anxiety of any patient is often revealed only when she is getting up to leave, so that again a barrier to useful work is created by the very situation. One woman kept a busy doctor fidgeting impatiently with hesitant, irrelevant questions for twenty minutes. She then rose saying, 'I must not keep you any longer. I have to get down to the hospital. My sister has cancer, but I understand it doesn't run in families.' Another irritated her doctor by the hysterical flippancy with which she discussed her recent secondary frigidity. Only at the door did she confess that her mother had died in a mental hospital at just her own age. Happily, the doctor had the wit to bring her back and allow the real underlying terror and misery to be wept through. The guilt that she had not paid more heed to her mother's difficulties at a time when she was only concerned with her own rich new sexual life was aired.

The fear of madness did indeed underlie her sudden need to control her sexual feelings.

We see these last-minute communications as indications of panic and desperation; as an accurate measure of the patient's difficulty in admitting her anxiety.

CHAPTER 6

The Presented Symptom

The heading is not a misprint. We have noted that many 'presenting' symptoms are never put into words. We study here the symptoms that many patients choose to present as a guise for the true problem, sexual difficulty, which it is more difficult for them to express. The choice of symptom is so often, when all is revealed, directly related to the nature of the inner difficulty, that it may provide an accurate focus for therapy.

We have to note that many women may use physical symptoms as respectable pretexts for seeking advice, but that this may also sometimes indicate that the patient needs to see her difficulties as physical, since to see them as emotional – as in her deeper self – is less tolerable than to be able to blame a bodily accident.

We note too that when a woman speaks of her vagina, her 'inside', she may often unconsciously be speaking also of her 'inside' feelings, hidden from the outside world and from the surface of her consciousness as her vagina is hidden from the surface of her body.

A patient complained of vaginal discharge. She was aloof and abrupt in manner, and adducted her knees firmly when examination was attempted. She thus made difficult exploration of both her body and her feelings. Interpretations eventually allowed both. Her discharge was negligible and frigidity was the real problem. It was necessary to explore her internalized parental prohibitions on sexuality. She saw her genitals as dirty and nasty and also as shameful and to be hidden. She felt the same about her sexual desires. When all was known, therefore, her presented symptom (a vagina dirty and concealed) and her demeanour (feelings to be concealed also) were directly related to the nature of her frigidity. It was possible to put her in touch with the excitement underlying these prohibitions and she was then able to enjoy her feelings in intercourse, and her vagina, in the 'cure' of her complaint of discharge.

A patient, therefore, who complains of discharge when there is very little, who asks for a smear or expresses a fear of cancer when it is improbable, or who worries about VD when she is unlikely to have been at risk, may well be expressing the feeling that there is something dirty or nasty about her vagina and about her sexual desires. Occasionally a patient who apologizes for a nonexistent mess or smell before examination, or who apologizes for coming straight from work or for not having bathed, may reveal the same difficulty. Others may alert the doctor to this situation without being able to express it verbally by excessive fastidiousness over underwear, pubic shaving, or 'feminine deodorants'. It is worth noting here also how some women vary in their reaction to examination if menstruating. While some do not mind at all, others obviously find the idea so repulsive as to be out of the question. The doctor's own attitude can be important here. Whether or not she in fact proceeds with the examination, it may be better to air the difficulty. To accept that examination is impossible may be to collude with, and thus reinforce, the patient's feeling of disgust. It is interesting, too, how many patients, having waited weeks or months to come, contrive to do so when menstruating and then expect to avoid examination. This may be a measure of their difficulty in allowing exploration of this, to them, disturbing area of body and feeling.

The complaint of dyspareunia may also be a way of saying 'It is not I, the person, who has sexual difficulties, it is just my body.' While fears of pain are often associated with fantasies of damage and rape, we have met cases in which the complaint of pain at intercourse meant very different things.

A young woman complained that intercourse had been increasingly painful since her marriage one year earlier, despite an extensive hymenectomy and vaginal repair. Her story of incipient depression – exhaustion, irritability, and social withdrawal – was at odds with her lively and cheerful appearance. Her life as an adopted daughter was recounted as happy and faultless, although exploration of her feelings about her adoptive parents led to speculation about her true origins, and she admitted to being haunted by a fear of death. All this made the doctor consider psychiatric referral.

However, the discussion of cap-fitting revealed a very different story. The patient admitted her longing for a baby. Coitus interruptus was practised and the 'pain' on intercourse came in fact after withdrawal. Interpretation that this was an emotional 'pain' enabled her to discuss her resentments of her husband for keeping his seed from her. Her depression was relieved and she soon returned, pregnant and delighted. The doctor was a little disappointed that, though the 'dyspareunia' was cured, the patient seemed indifferent to the idea of wishing to enjoy intercourse for its own sake. It may be that there was a parallel between the feeling of withdrawal in intercourse and the 'withdrawal' of her true parents from her life, and that her capacity to relate deeply required further interpretations, which were at this stage too difficult for her to face.

29

We meet patients who have been fully investigated for sub-fertility without physical cause being detected, and who in answer to a straight question have said that intercourse is all right. For many, the importance of conceiving undoubtedly causes stresses in love-making that has to be by the calendar. It is not unusual to find vaginismus at a post-coital test, or indeed spasm at tubal insufflation, which relaxes in response to interpretation of this stress. This often accounts for the common finding that subfertile couples conceive after adoption proceedings have been instituted and they can revert to making love when they feel like it, rather than for the one purpose of conception.

With other patients, however, who seem very insistent that the cause must be physical, even though none has been found, the interpretation that it is difficult for them to admit that feelings might be involved may produce surprising material.

One patient who complained of subfertility and insisted that she knew all about the facts of conception, brandished textbooks of physiology and perfect basal temperature charts. On the couch, however, she admitted that she and her husband only made love about once in two months and rarely at the fertile times. Intercourse for its own sake was unimportant to her; the cultural interests that they shared were so much more rewarding. Exploration revealed parents with high academic aspirations for her, who opposed boy-friends until she had graduated. She had felt it necessary to be adult, brainy, and sensible before her time in order to earn their approval, and unsexy too, of course. It was possible to put her in touch with her needs to have not only sexiness but also babyishness approved. With the doctor's approval she was able to learn to value her own babyish needs and also to lift her internal ban on sexual desire. This patient who had come complaining of subfertility left with a cap saying that she wanted time to enjoy her sexual life first. She did later conceive and bear two lovely children and showed no desire to return to her academic career until they 'had less need of her', because she 'could not bear to miss their cuddly stage'. The baby she was apparently seeking was the baby inside herself.

Problems attributed to different contraceptive methods deserve a chapter to themselves, since these are the group most commonly encountered in family-planning practice. It is worth noting here the patient who insists that all is well in this respect, but in fact finds other symptoms to draw attention to herself while disguising that she has an emotional problem.

A patient attended for a year for her pills, and had attended for a cap for two years previously. During this time she had become friends with many members of the clinic staff by her gay helpful manner, and the doctor always found her quite charming. They would discuss their children together, and the local arts club, in which both were interested. It took these three years for the doctor to notice that, although clinically 'everything was fine', the patient had tried three different caps and three changes of pill. Always it was, 'Yes, it suits me beautifully, it's just that I have these blinding headaches' or 'this continual bleeding'. Her inability to complain and be an ordinary patient was the measure of her difficulty in owning to needs or problems. When the doctor finally observed that no method they tried seemed very satisfactory but that she did not seem to dare to complain, the patient could angrily reveal her resentment that her husband no longer had the responsibility. Intercourse could then be discussed more freely, and the patient could tearfully admit that she had found his sperm messy and distasteful. With the sheath and coitus interruptus she had been spared this and had enjoyed intercourse to the full; with female methods she hated it. To her, intercourse, both sexual and social, needed to be 'nice' – all sweetness and light. Put in touch with the underlying

31

excitement in this concept of 'nasty mess', the patient was able to reach orgasm again without reverting to male methods.

Finally, we need to notice that the presented symptom may be something outside the patient altogether, namely the husband. Many women come to the clinic saying in effect, 'There is nothing the matter with me but my husband unfortunately has premature ejaculation – or is too slow, or too eager or not eager enough.' We find it very difficult with such patients not to send the husband, whom we have never met, for treatment, and to recognize that the patient is the one who comes. Yet to do so is to collude with, and to reinforce, the woman's need to believe that her feelings are not involved, and her fear that there is nothing she can or should wish to do to help.

Again, we should keep calm and notice how the patient is getting us to behave. From this we may gain insight into the situation the husband faces with the same woman.

A pretty young woman came, as some do, with a metaphorical shopping-list for the doctor about which methods she would or would not consider, saying that she had to take charge (at home, as well as at the clinic!) because her husband had premature ejaculation. The doctor, who had already found herself bursting in precipitously when the patient drew breath, felt some sympathetic identification with him. She could interpret the patient's need to be in charge – of something in herself too, perhaps. It was revealed that she had had wonderful wild-animal feelings about intercourse with a previous boy-friend. Instead of taking this at its face value as confirmation of the patient's own sexual talent and therefore of the husband's inadequacies, the doctor observed that she had in fact fled from this exciting affair and chosen instead her 'safe' husband, whom she described as rather dull – 'an ideal family man'.

The patient was then able to discuss her strict convent upbringing and her parents: her intellectual mother who never discussed sex, on the one hand; her exciting earthy father, whose sheaths she would secretly count in the bathroom to know when her parents had had intercourse, on the other. These two bits of herself were examined and understood. Earthy, sexy, excited by men – this was bad, and unfaithful to mother. After a summer holiday in which intercourse was 'marvellous' (notice this untreated husband's remarkable recovery!), the patient was transformed in appearance and attitude – calm, responsive and radiant. They were moving into a new house and lining it with carpets, giving the doctor the impression of a cosy fur-lined nest, and she could see that her mother and the convent were not right. Sex and brains could mix (a tribute to the doctor perhaps) and they were moving to another town to 'live our own lives'.

Other patients seem to project their own attitudes to sexuality on to their husbands, and there find them unsatisfactory. The patient who says, 'He wants it all the time, isn't it awful?' may well be testing against the doctor her own feeling of the awfulness of her own desires. The doctor who identifies in sympathy with the 'awfulness' thereby confirms the patient's feeling that she has no business to own such desires.

Another patient who, on the face of it, was married to the wrong man, was enabled to find the exciting male in the husband she had. Despite a teasing, provocative manner, she said she was contemplating divorce because she was completely uninterested in sex and they did not have intercourse any more. She never had been interested in sex, but expected that 'although it would be painful it would be wonderful'. With two tough, exciting previous boy-friends, she had allowed heavy petting but had always managed to

D   33 defeat them over intercourse – 'just!' she twinkled. She went on to describe her husband most contemptuously as dull, obedient to her every whim, gentle; and to say that when he meekly did foolish menial tasks to please her she wanted to throw something. He had once shown some spark under provocation, and had nearly smashed a valuable glass vase. Her disappointment that he had not done so was evident and could be interpreted in terms of her disappointment with his gentle sexual techniques. The symbolism of smashing glass, as in the Jewish marriage ceremony and many other customs and rituals, is another that may often be fruitfully interpreted in this work. The teasing quality of this patient was paralleled in examination when she asked for a cap, and then said there was no point because they did not have intercourse.

Put in touch with her own provocation and pulling back, her need to have her protestations overcome, to put up a sexual fight and be sure of losing it, this patient came back saying that her husband was more co-operative, but, more important, so was she. She thought perhaps they might start a family. A year later the doctor received a bunch of flowers and a letter saying all was wonderful and they were so grateful. They had moved into a lovely new house (*sic*) and were expecting their first baby with great pleasure.

Now that the treatment of marital difficulties is more widely advertised at FPA clinics, some male patients do come or are referred in their own right. The psychophysical technique here described is not found to be of particular value in the treatment of male psychosexual difficulties. It seems that, unlike the vagina, the penis is from the earliest years an organ whose structure, purpose, and pleasure potential are obvious. The fantasy-versus-fact confrontation, so useful in examination of the female genitals, therefore carries no dramatic revelation of insight for the male. Such useful treatment as we can achieve with shaky potency or premature ejaculation when the man himself is the *a priori* patient, is based upon techniques which are psychotherapeutic rather than psycho-physical. Such techniques are not the subject of this book or of this training; but to learn, as we do, that aggressive and awkward people can be seen, not as wicked or stupid but rather as frightened or troubled, cannot fail to improve our dealings with anxious patients of either sex.

We can report, therefore, only on the difficulties of those men whose wives or girl-friends we treat, and not on those who seek help elsewhere for themselves. Of those male problems we do meet at secondhand in this way – premature ejaculation and impotence – we can say confidently that the commonest cause is frigidity in the partner; and that success-ful treatment of that frigidity will cure the secondary male difficulty without the need to see the man.

CHAPTER 7

Unconscious Factors and
Contraceptive Methods

Few medical topics have received such world-wide, large-scale statistical study as the relative efficiency of contraceptive methods. It is inevitable, however, that such studies are based upon the assumption that the patient is merely a physical body governed by a wholly rational mind, and that the doctor is making equally objective physical and rational observations. It is not our task to question such figures. They are crucial – other things being equal – to the quality of advice we may give our patients.

However, it is important to recognize that when the measuring instrument – the doctor – is equipped to observe unconscious factors, surprisingly different results may be obtained. This crucial variable we have found to affect significantly in many cases the motivation to contraceptive effort, the choice of method, and the efficiency with which the given patient is able to use such methods. We have found too that insistence upon, or rejection of, or difficulty with, a particular method may be yet another way in which a patient may reveal underlying sexual anxiety. Some examples of these situations are discussed in this chapter.

36

Motivation to Contraceptive Methods

Patients who feel unconsciously that the right purpose of intercourse is conception may find difficulties with any serious contraceptive effort. A woman complained of loss of orgasm with the cap. Examination revealed that she also had no enthusiasm when the sheath had been used previously, and that she could now only tolerate intercourse at about the time of ovulation. Suggestions that the pill might be better for her produced the reaction, 'It is too safe.' She revealed that she had only enjoyed intercourse to the full when they were trying for each of her three children. She had on each occasion found orgasm impossible after her first missed period until she had finished feeding each of the babies. Her own mother had been very close and protective to each of her own three children, but the patient had the impression from her that sex for its own sake was an improper and prohibited desire. Interpretation of these difficulties enabled the patient to begin to enjoy intercourse again, regardless of the method chosen.

A similar emotional pattern may directly affect the efficiency of a particular method. Another woman, an efficient atheist mathematician, was constantly changing her mind about taking the pill, and was thus frequently at risk through irregular cycles and medications. This behaviour seemed totally at odds with the rational competent image she presented. Exploration revealed a childhood with parents always abroad and a deep feeling for the values of the nuns who taught her and provided her closest loving relationships. Intellectually she totally rejected Roman Catholicism; yet emotionally each renewed religious controversy brought to the surface unconscious doubts about the rightness of her sexual desires while using contraception. Interpretation brought her to terms with this, and she was able to enjoy intercourse and take the pill efficiently.

Similarly, a combined pill eventually failed a woman who, each time she was frightened by a press report of thrombo-embolism, would 'forget' to take several pills.

Choice of Method

Difficulties may arise for women who begin to take responsi-bility for the contraceptive method, whichever female method is chosen. Two such patterns of emotional difficulty, which often occur separately, were involved with the patient referred to in the previous chapter, who had difficulty once she had to take this responsibility. One was the distasteful excitement and associated resentments at receiving sperm. We meet many patients who confess to this in the context of a doctor–patient relationship that allows discussion of what is to them a very delicate and embarrassing matter. Another patient, in middle age, going on the pill for maximum efficiency, found that the orgasm she had regularly achieved with coitus interruptus was lost with the pill. Many patients complain of lack of enthusiasm with the pill, and early in the study most of the doctors felt that the explanation was hor-monal in nearly all cases. With increasing experience in exploration of the patient's feelings, we now find that 'hormonal frigidity', which does seem occasionally to occur despite deep scrutiny, is the exception rather than the rule.

In the case of the middle-aged patient, a clue to the idea that the obvious hormonal explanation would not suffice was detected in the fact that she implied the doctor should suggest to her husband that they should 'ease up' at their age. She revealed great unease about her own sexual excitement now that her children were reaching sexual maturity. The maxi-mum efficiency offered by the pill was vital to her lest preg-nancy should reveal that she still had a sexual life. But her husband's emission inside her, never before experienced, was too exciting. Her mounting feelings were switched off in panic at their height, leaving her with disappointment and frustration, which she reported as 'disgust'. Interpretation of her need for permission still to enjoy her sexual life was sufficient for her to resume orgasm despite the pill. Incidentally, she changed in appearance from a rather scruffy, depressed middle-aged frump into a well-groomed, cheerful person looking ten years younger. She took a part-time job to help pay for redecorating the house; her relationships were transformed, not only with her husband but with her teenage daughter who had had behaviour problems. The mother no longer resented her emerging sexuality, and the girl's school performance improved.

This patient had also resented having to take control and responsibility. A similar pattern frequently appears when a change from male to female methods is undertaken for added efficiency. Another woman had enjoyed a rich and joyful marriage with three babies planned successfully with the sheath and vaginal orgasm nearly every time. An obstetric difficulty prompted the necessity for maximum efficiency – the combined pill. From that moment she had no orgasm and her eagerness for intercourse had rapidly dwindled until after nine months it was nonexistent. Inquiries about feeling the risk of pregnancy to be important to her drew a blank, as did various changes of prescription. Eventually the doctor noticed that she was having to make all the suggestions without co-operation, and related this to the way the patient spoke of her once so splendid husband. He had been ill, demoted at work, and was no help around the house. Interpretation of this resentment enabled the patient to admit her difficulty in taking responsibility – for practical decisions about the family and contraception, and for her own sexual desires also. The pill, simple and unpremeditated though it is, was enough to make her feel too responsible for intercourse. She had grown up with the idea that sex was for men. When her husband was in charge with the sheath, she could respond to the full, as it were despite herself. With the idea that she was entitled to pleasure for her own sake out in the open, she was able to resume orgasm. Her husband soon found a better job under the influence of her return to sexual responsiveness!

We have referred before to the patient with cap difficulties, who has difficulty in accepting her vagina and touching it and also in accepting her own sexual desires. Such patients often get pregnant with the cap, not because it is ill-fitting or because they are technically incapable of using it, but because they find it distasteful and therefore keep it in the bathroom cupboard rather than in their vagina. Interpretations of the emotions underlying distaste or difficulty are therefore vital at the time of fitting if the cap is to be efficient. Similar emotional patterns are often encountered with patients who refuse an intra-uterine device on the ground that they do not like to think of having 'something inside', and with those who insist that the pill is the only method for them. It is worth noting that many patients who ask for a change to the pill expect in it a magical cure for their sexual difficulties. While in many cases the absolute certainty of the pill may help for a few months, it is our experience that where the underlying difficulty is not fear of pregnancy *per se*, but rather a more complex emotional one, the magical cure rarely lasts. We have come to describe the type that conforms to this pattern as the 'no-touch patient'. Young patients, and premaritals particularly, who insist that only the pill will do alert us to the possibility of difficulties with the vagina and with vaginal feeling. There are twofold merits in interpretation in this situation. A young girl with many years ahead of potential risk may be persuaded to accept the cap for a time and may also be helped to explore and accept her vagina and its feelings by self-examination even if the pill is finally to be the chosen method. Fears and disappointments about intercourse may be explored, and the patient helped towards consummation and orgasm.

In the matter of choice of method too, therefore, it is often the case that the presented difficulty may be directly related to the nature of the problem. An exaggerated instance of reluctance to take responsibility for intercourse, for contraception, and for her own desires, is sometimes met with in the patient who insists upon an IUD. With this method, of course, the patient literally has to do nothing for herself. The device is inserted by someone else and she does not have to think about it at all. We have met patients like this who refuse to take responsibility in other aspects of their life. Often the doctor finds herself having to do all the work without any response from the patient, and is not surprised to hear that the husband at home is put in the same position. While the IUD does, of course, in many cases cause heavy and painful periods or intermenstrual spotting for purely physical reasons, it is noteworthy that patients vary very much in their reaction to this, as they do in their reaction to the side-effects of other methods. There are patients who will willingly put up with these difficulties for the contraceptive benefits they confer. Others may complain bitterly about their heavy and painful periods with the loop, and in response to sensitive interpretation may reveal the resentments they feel about their responsibility for intercourse. Again, it is not surprising that a woman who sees intercourse as for her husband's pleasure alone, and who resents this, is more likely to 'suffer' from side-effects than one who can see such methods as a small price to pay for her own pleasure and fulfilment.

We have met patients too who blame the sheath for their lack of enjoyment, and who on further examination blame their husbands. The idea that they could do something about intercourse in order to make it better was foreign to them. They needed to see the difficulty as outside themselves. It is important here to comment upon the concept of 'penis-envy' – Freud's name for the complex in which a woman resents manhood and the penis, feeling it to be something she lacks. We have met this frequently and have come to see it in many cases not as a primary difficulty but rather as a defensive system against a deeper difficulty about the implications of being a woman (see Chapter 9).

A patient who appeared rather tough and matter-of-fact revealed resentments of her husband's orgasm, which she saw as better than her own. She complained also that she wished he would spend more time on her and less upon his car, and was able to accept the interpretation that she felt the same about his technique in intercourse. To the interpretation that she seemed to feel that men always had the best of it, the patient responded that she had always been a tomboy as a child, feeling boys' toys and games to be more exciting than girls'. She believed that her parents had really wanted a boy rather than a girl. The doctor went on to put her in touch with the idea that a woman was a good and valuable thing to be in its own right, and the patient began to understand why she valued herself, her feelings, and her vagina so little. She began to dress and behave in a more feminine fashion, and to see her vagina not as a poor substitute for a penis but as a valid organ of feeling in its own right. Her fantasy was that feminine feeling, if uncontrolled, would be foolish, laughable, and vulnerable. To see that a competent adult – the doctor – could value such foolish, laughable, and vulnerable aspects of herself was enough to give her confidence to show these same aspects to her husband in intercourse, abandoning those defensive control systems which are so fatal to the achievement of feminine orgasm.

CHAPTER 8

Virginal Anxiety

At the start of our study of the female contribution to unconsummated marriages, we had the benefit of the recent publica-
tion of the report of the original FPA group's findings.[1] From
it there emerged for us various foci of special study. I shall not
reiterate its material here. *Virgin Wives*, with Dr Balint's book
on the doctor–patient relationship,[2] should be read by everyone seriously interested in the present subject. I therefore
merely emphasize here that in studying our doctor–patient
relationships, we too encountered the maternally enjoined
'innocence' of the 'sleeping beauty'; the defensive–aggressive,
destructive 'Brunhild'; and the 'queen bee', wishing for virgin
motherhood. We, like our colleagues, however, found such
clear-cut classification rare and difficult. We, like them, found
more often that these attitudes blurred and overlapped in
different patients who would show facets of several patterns.

Having noted their interest in the importance of the
physical transactions of their clinic gynaecology, we studied
with special emphasis the emotional communications offered
or concealed by patients at these moments. In so doing we

---

[1] Leonard J. Friedman, *Virgin Wives*. Mind and Medicine Monographs,
London: Tavistock; Philadelphia and Toronto: Lippincott, 1962.
[2] Michael Balint, *The Doctor, his Patient and the Illness*. London: Pitman;
New York: International Universities Press, 1957.

believe we can throw added light on the nature of the non-consummation difficulty and on the nature of the mechanism by which we are able to help its resolution.

In addition, we made a special study of premarital patients. Those who were already having intercourse have been discussed earlier (Chapter 5). Among those premarital patients who came before intercourse had either been achieved or attempted, we found many who revealed anxieties, fantasies, and personality patterns of startling similarity to those encountered in unconsummated marriages. It seems reasonable, therefore, to regard this as one clinical complex which I describe as 'virginal anxiety', in which married and unmarried are distinguished by their legal status rather than by their emotional attitude. Patients do, of course, have an emotional attitude towards the legal status itself. Some implications of this are discussed in the next chapter.

Parental Prohibition

One of the commonest situations encountered, not only in virginal anxiety but in frigidity also, is that implied in Friedman's concept of the 'sleeping beauty', who could not allow herself to be sexually awakened until her prohibitive parents were figuratively dead. The patient feels that her parents, usually her mother, have not given her permissive encouragement to own her own sexuality – her vagina, her desires, or her feelings of womanhood. These still emotionally belong to her mother and cannot be faced or used without guilt. The guilt may be about the infidelity to the father implied in relating to another man, or about treachery to the mother in wishing for a man of her own when 'man' belongs to the mother. More often, however, in our field, the patient's uneasiness is that to be sexy is to be the sort of person her mother disapproves of. It will be seen, therefore, that with such patients the emphasis is on parental relationships; that is, they are still more daughters than lovers or wives.

The situation may be presented by patients in a variety of ways. They may say 'mother never told me about sex', or that they had to learn it from books, or schoolfriends, or dirty jokes, or that menstruation or their own desires took them, in their innocence, by surprise; or that they never talked or even thought about sex. Conversely, some say that their parents were very free and frank, but that they felt that it was only for them – the parents – and did not apply to themselves. The hint is thus raised that something in the patient may need such positive encouragement; that whatever her parents' actual attitude, she cannot, as it were, grant such permission or accept it internally for herself.

One has, of course, the opportunity of discussing parental attitudes with many patients who have no difficulty in using their sexuality with freedom, and whom in this context we may call 'non-patients'. Without having accurate comparative figures, the overwhelming clinical impression is that the range of actual parental attitudes is equally varied and comparable between the two groups – patients and non-patients. If this is true, it confirms the hint that actual parental action signifies less than the individual patient's capacity to accept or reject their attitudes without guilt. This is not to dismiss the parents from the scene, since clearly the individual patient's capacity must stem from them in some degree, but perhaps at an earlier and more primitive level than that of sex education. The matter has, however, technical importance in the clinical treatment of these problems.

If the doctor accepts the patient's interpretation of her parents' attitude as *de facto*, then deep and possibly prolonged exploration of early relationships is necessary, and may well prove beyond the scope of the psychophysical doctor. It is possible, however, to respond to these communications about parental attitudes with an observation such as, 'Anyhow, this is how it seemed to you.' The treatment is then focused back to the patient's own reaction and to the here-and-now doctor–patient relationship, in which the patient's own

45

difficulty in accepting sexuality for herself may be directly examined.

Having done this, we have studied how the process of encouraging the patient to touch, explore, and feel with her vagina has such dramatic therapeutic effect. Having seen for herself that she has needed such permission and encouragement because of her inability to grasp her own womanhood, the patient finds herself able to accept it for herself from the doctor, a mother-substitute, recognizing that, as a woman, her own mother's actual attitude need no longer inhibit her from within her own feelings.

Fact and Fantasy

In focusing our attention on the emotional attitudes of the patient towards vaginal examination, we have encountered a large group who, in contrast to those just discussed whom one may call the 'innocent', may be described as the 'ignorant'. Many patients with virginal anxiety cannot allow themselves to know or to speculate about how their vaginae are made, what their sexual sensations will be like, or how the first intercourse will be. The commonest fantasy first encountered was that the entrance or the passage itself was too small. Associated with it was the idea that the sexy woman in the patient was a too-small part of herself, and the fantasy that intercourse itself, and in parallel her own feelings about it, would be dangerous, painful, and traumatic. Such patients have been helped to express fears of intolerable pain, of massive haemorrhage, or of being literally torn apart, or that the penis will 'break through' into some wrong and fearful place such as the rectum or the womb itself or the abdominal cavity. In parallel with these physical fears is the fear that intercourse will 'break through' into some unspeakable part of the patient's feelings, and that loss of control here will make of her a frighteningly different person.

It is important to recognize that, as was stressed in Chapter

3, intellectual factual knowledge to the contrary is not enough to dispel these unconscious anxieties. We encountered a biology graduate who revealed her fantasy that there was only one passage, the urethra, through which the penis must force its way into a kind of cloaca. Logically this patient had only to refer to her textbooks to realize the fallacy. However, she had suffered repeated painful catheterizations in childhood, so that her fears of pain in intercourse were not hard to imagine in unconscious terms. Other patients have feared that the vagina leads to a vast cavern the size of a full-term fundus, so that things may be lost in or damaged by it.

We have met many patients whose first treatment for their inability to consummate was surgery. Some had also been fully stretched by dilators after hymenectomy or vaginal repair. Despite the rational knowledge thus produced that they were large enough physically, many were still unable to allow penetration, and insisted that there was still a wall to be broken through. Reassurance and the encouragement to explore were in these cases never enough unless the underlying fantasy was fully aired. For these patients the first intercourse had to be painful or disturbing, if not physically then emotionally, and the clinical anaesthetized adjustments simply did not fulfil the expected experience of breaking through the emotional 'wall'. It is usual to find here the expectation of a raping experience, and it is necessary to put the patient in touch with the excitement underlying the fear. The patient can then recognize that the emotional 'break-through' will indeed be to a different, disturbing, exciting part of her emotional self. In such cases the psycho-physical technique now operates on a different and dual mechanism. First, the frightening fantasy of damage and pain is confronted by the fact of a vagina, which the patient can explore with her fingers and find to be different – larger, more elastic, with sound protective walls or whatever. In parallel, the doctor in her encouragement is implying emotionally that the new person and her desires and excitement are something good and to be wished for, rather than frightening and to be controlled. Is it so terrible to be this kind of person with wishes of this kind? One apparently respectable adult, the doctor, having heard 'the worst', thinks not.

CHAPTER 9

Conditional Frigidity

In this work we define frigidity as the inability to achieve vaginal orgasm within the act of intercourse, that is with the penis in the vagina. We consider as frigid patients those who are unable to achieve this and who in one way or another express the wish to do so, or feel that their sexual life lacks this final culmination.

Before discussing in the final chapter the understanding and treatment of women who have never been able to achieve this, comment is required about our findings in many women with less total disability. We meet many women who have in the past been able to achieve full mutual vaginal orgasm in intercourse, but who have lost this ability. This situation may be described as secondary frigidity. Others can achieve orgasm only in certain circumstances, or only by other means than within the act of intercourse itself.

The means to orgasm is, of course, largely a matter of personal taste or choice, and many women who, for example, obtain their satisfaction through clitoral stimulation either before or after penetration are happy this way. However, there are very many also who complain to us that this is not, they feel, all they had hoped, and who would like to change. This we describe as conditional or qualified frigidity.

Secondary Frigidity

It is not unusual – perhaps hardly pathological – for young women new to motherhood to find the emotional demands of the baby pushing aside to some degree their sexual desire for their husband. Disastrous though this may be to the marital relationship and to the father–child relationship if real rejection persists, the situation is often so obvious that the simplest interpretation is enough to improve the wife's response. We do meet, however, many women whose frigidity after childbirth is more deep-seated and more serious.

Sometimes psycho-physical interpretation of her changed feelings about her vagina is necessary. One young woman complained that since her forceps delivery any attempt at intercourse had been too 'painful'. The baby was now six months old, and in fact it became clear that nothing even approaching penetration had been allowed. On examination there was adduction of the knees, but the perineum was well healed and no tenderness was detected. The patient confessed tearfully that she thought that she would 'never be the same again'. The difficult birth and suturing in the lithotomy position she had felt to be humiliating in its exposure and its messiness. She could no longer bear to think of the vagina herself, or of sharing it. Simple interpretation and encouragement to explore the now healed, clean and 'lovable' vagina were enough to allow her to resume intercourse with pleasure and orgasm. This case might thus be regarded as one of secondary nonconsummation.

For other patients the factor of maternal prohibition seems to arise for the first time after a change of circumstances.

After childbirth the patient, now a mother, is unable to enjoy her previously lively sexuality on the unconscious ground that 'mothers don't do it'. Because of her feeling about her mother's attitude to sex, she finds that while she could achieve orgasm as a rebellious young lover, the fact of motherhood prohibits this. Again exploration and interpretation with encouragement and 'permission' enable her to question whether she herself needs to be this kind of non-sexual mother, and she is able to resume orgasm.

A patient came for the pill, hoping that it might improve her sexual life, since she had been unable to achieve orgasm since the birth of her second child. Previously she had enjoyed intercourse to the full with a cap, for some eight years, so that the doctor was able to dismiss at once the question of contraceptive method as a wish for magical help and a pretext for coming, and get down to the exploration of the change in her feelings. The patient had been tomboyish in childhood, intolerant of silly girlish things, and her mother had said that she could be feminine but not in an obvious way. She could accept the doctor's interpretation that perhaps she could be motherly but not sexy, and was able to discuss her difficulties with tenderness. She worried about her baby, but was unable to cuddle him. She presented as jolly and hearty, and the doctor was able to show her that this tomboyish heartiness was a defence system against her fears of foolish girlish tenderness. She could see that this interpretation of her mother's attitude, valuing boyish commonsense and sensible motherhood, but not foolish girlish tenderness, had been internalized within her. She returned looking more feminine with a new fluffy hairstyle and pretty clothes, her sexual life already improving.

It is interesting that marriage itself is often the precipitating factor of secondary frigidity on the basis of 'mother must not know'. Some patients who have been able to enjoy full orgasm before marriage, when it was secret, are unable to respond equally after the wedding. The simple interpretation of forbidden fruit may not be sufficient unless the patient can see that she has internalized respectable prohibitions on sexual

51

desire. One such patient said that she had enjoyed vaginal orgasm regularly during courtship, despite the sheath and despite the fact that they were in her parents' living-room and had to be careful that the parents did not come home unexpectedly early and catch them. She had expected that after marriage everything would be idyllic in their own home, but had suddenly felt at the white wedding her mother had arranged 'the declaring in the face of this congregation that this is what we are going to do'. From that moment she 'froze', feeling that everyone knew each time they had intercourse. Again, simple interpretation and permissive encouragement from a different kind of doctor–mother was sufficient for orgasm to be resumed.

Another patient complained that she could no longer enjoy intercourse in marriage because of the fear of pregnancy. This seemed illogical since the fear of pregnancy would presumably have been greater before marriage. It emerged that she had conceived and had an abortion, although she 'would have loved to have the baby', on the grounds that 'everyone would know' (that they were having intercourse), and that her mother would be terribly hurt by the premature pregnancy because she had taught her that 'good girls wait'. Even after marriage, the patient now felt that pregnancy would reveal to the world, and to her mother in particular, that she was having intercourse. Rationally, of course, her mother would expect her to after marriage. What this patient feared was her mother's reaction to the fact that this was the sort of girl her daughter was – a girl with sexual desires that should not be admitted, licensed or no.

Other patients who become frigid after termination of pregnancy seem to be punishing themselves for the wicked consequences of their pleasure and orgasm by clamping down on their sexual desires.

One young woman was still living with the boy-friend who had fathered her child and they were planning to marry 'sometime'. She had had a backstreet abortion in panic about what 'people' (parents) would say, although at that time she was having regular orgasms, they were very much in love, and were planning to marry soon. Since the abortion, which she felt was 'terrible – sordid, shameful, but what I deserved', she was taking the pill, sleeping with her boy-friend, but having intercourse only rarely and then without any sensation for her. The marriage had been postponed indefinitely – 'until I feel certain of my feelings again'. This patient is to date unable to respond to permissive encouragement although she is able to accept the interpretation that she is punishing herself for her early sexuality and the abortion. The 'child' she feels she has destroyed is the child in herself.

Another woman, married, had enjoyed intercourse to the full until the very necessary termination of her third pregnancy on life-saving medical grounds. She had felt since, although it was not her own wish, that accepting the advice to terminate was 'the most evil thing I ever did'. She can now only allow herself any feeling in intercourse when she feels there is a slight chance of pregnancy, even though medically she knows that such a pregnancy would be disastrous. Not surprisingly, exploration revealed that this patient had felt herself to be an unwanted child. She was in need of deeper psychotherapy and interpretation, and psycho-physical encouragement was insufficient for the resumption of sexual pleasure.

It is an important part of seminar training to recognize the differential diagnosis of patients whose problems are too deep-seated for treatment by these methods in short-term clinic visits. Special sessions are available in many FPA centres for patients requiring long-term exploration, but for other patients their sexual difficulty is only the presenting symptom in a deeper psychological illness or personality disorder. Then psychiatric referral is, of course, necessary. A patient may, for example, become depressed as a result of her marital difficulties, and when the marital difficulties are relieved the depression is cured. Equally, however, a patient suffering from endogenous depression may present with frigidity and the exploration of her sexual attitudes may do more harm than good. There is no substitute for clinical experience in deciding these matters, but seminar training does go far towards improving diagnostic skills in this respect.

'Clitoral' Orgasm – The Real Thing?

We have discussed earlier how some patients' capacity for orgasm seems before therapy to depend upon, for example, one method of contraception or another, or upon whether they are trying for a pregnancy. For many patients orgasm is easy by clitoral stimulation, but they feel something is missing or that this is not the real thing. The penis in the vagina does not however for them produce a sensation that leads to orgasm, or they feel there is no feeling there at all, or their desire and excitement are 'switched off' at the moment of penetration.

Masters and Johnson[1] have shown with apparent conclusiveness that, in physical terms, vaginal orgasm is produced by the stimulation of the clitoris by the action of the penis. We can say confidently, however, that, in emotional terms, stimulation of the clitoris by petting and the orgasm thus produced is a different experience psychically from the experience of orgasm with the penis in the vagina. The togetherness, mutual abandonment of control systems, the emotional acceptance of the penis and all it implies in terms of the man, and of the vagina and all it implies in terms of the woman, make this a unique experience that is not mimicked emotionally by mutual masturbation however loving. It is emotionally

[1] W. H. Masters and V. E. Johnson, *Human Sexual Response*, Boston: Little Brown; Churchill, 1966.

more difficult for many people, and many who cannot achieve it know that they are missing something. Equally, many who can achieve it are in no doubt as to its importance or as to the difference.

We find that in many cases putting a woman who has hitherto only enjoyed orgasm through the clitoris in touch with her vaginal sensation through our well-tried psychophysical techniques may be very useful. One often finds the opportunity to draw attention to the emotional/physical parallel in that, as her sensation is chiefly on the outside, so may her sexual feelings be chiefly superficial also. Clitoral sensation is usually experienced and learned early, be the pleasure thus discovered guilt-ridden or no. Vaginal sensation (or perhaps we should say, since Masters and Johnson, 'intercourse sensation') does need to some extent to be learned to be appreciated, even in the absence of emotional prohibition. Having recognized her difficulties and shared them with the doctor, a woman will, in coming to accept for herself the concept of the vagina as a touchable acceptable organ of pleasure also come to accept its sensations and her own desires as permissible and exciting.

However, often in patients who complain that orgasm can be by digital stimulation of the clitoris only, which must be by definition outside the act of intercourse itself, deeper difficulties are encountered. We often find the concept of penis-envy helpful to the understanding of such patients.

This concept, referred to in Chapter 7, implies a woman's feeling of being a second-class sex, lacking this brave organ, symbol and instrument of potent manhood, the penis. Unconsciously she envies man, the organ, and all it represents, and reacts against them with resentment, anger, and the need to control or to destroy. We have met patients who felt this way, and who, if not wholly frigid, have enjoyed only clitoral pleasure. Some have said they always felt a boy was a better thing to be than a girl, or that their parents always wanted a boy. Others have, in their aggressively controlling life-pattern,

55

like Brunhild, seen their love-life as a battle to be won, but have been saddened by the destructive effect of their winning. In the present context it seems that for them the separate, individual orgasm of mutual masturbation is easier than orgasm within intercourse. A little more of themselves is controlled and held back or, conversely a little more of the man is controlled and kept out. Orgasm within intercourse implies a total abandonment of these controls; a total acceptance not only of the vagina and of the female emotions associated with it, but also of the penis and all it emotionally implies in terms of the relationship to a man. The absence of this totality of sharing and mutual acceptance may have disastrous effects upon the relationship for many people. Husbands feel less than fully loved and accepted, while wives in their disappointment become resentful or blaming.

A young bride of eighteen months came for a cap-check and complained that she could not enjoy intercourse itself, having earlier enjoyed mutual masturbation to the full. She had now reached the state when she could not bear her husband to touch her at all. She confessed that she felt very masculine and was worried about homosexuality since she was becoming interested in the idea of men together, and was also obsessed by horror films and death, finding all these ideas both repugnant and fascinating. She felt her husband was defective in something which should stimulate her clitoris in intercourse, but hated the sensation of the penis inside. She had masturbated in adolescence and would have hated her mother to know – and yet would have liked to shock her.

This patient was extremely controlling in the interviews, but during interpretations was put in touch with the excitement underlying all these repugnant feelings. She began to complain less of her husband and to discuss the fears underlying the need to keep control. Her sexy, passionate feelings would shock people. The doctor was not shocked, and the patient could see that it was she herself who felt the idea as shocking. Then she was able to face the idea of how she might be really 'showing herself' in vaginal orgasm – violated, exposed, wide-open, and vulnerable. At the next visit vaginal orgasm had been achieved and the patient was radiant and delighted. Her husband, she confessed proudly, had danced round the room with delight, and she could confess that she had always found the penis exciting but had felt ashamed to admit it.

Another patient complained that she had enjoyed orgasm from petting before her marriage, and from masturbation, which she still practised, but since the wedding she had prevented her husband from touching her vulva because she wanted 'the real thing'. She felt no pleasure in intercourse, however, and found it difficult to allow penetration at all. She spoke disparagingly of her husband, reflecting savage contempt in masturbating after intercourse 'because she was bored'. The doctor commented upon this and interpreted it while paying tribute to her vagina during cap-fitting. The patient returned with enthusiasm and was able to discuss her fantasies of being chased nude through the woods and taken by storm. It became clear that she had felt it would be much better to be man and felt her parents had wished for her to be a boy. She admitted that the masturbation she had boasted of so freely had left her with deep feelings of shame. The fantasies of others having intercourse could give her an orgasm, and she preferred to be on top in intercourse herself, but felt this to be shameful. Intellectually this patient came to accept her vagina, her desires, and her womanhood, and lost her fears of becoming a man and her wishes to become a man. The marriage was consummated regularly, but vaginal orgasm was a rare exception. Emotionally the patient could not fully accept the doctor's evaluation of womanhood. She was frightened of being a woman, so fell back upon being a man.

For patients who feel that the penis is a necessary prerequisite of true sexual pleasure, the clitoris is indeed a poor substitute. We find that the necessary focus of therapy is once again the vagina; the exploration of the feeling of its inadequacy, or nastiness, or unimportance, or vulnerability; followed by the encouragement to value it not as a second-class substitute for a penis but as a valid organ of total feeling in its own right. In parallel with these bodily attitudes goes the emotional corollary. The idea that woman is the second-class sex, that female capacities and female desires are poor imitations of the male, is explored. The idea is then encouraged that to be a first-class woman is a richer and more fruitful aim than to be a second-class man.

An important conclusion has been suggested by Dr Main as the result of our consistent findings, and has been repeatedly confirmed in this study. The implication of Freud's work is that penis-envy is a primary difficulty. We have found consistently that the syndrome itself may be interpreted. The result of this interpretation is to reveal what to the patient is the primary difficulty in being a woman, the many facets of which are discussed in the final chapter. It is our conclusion, therefore, that penis-envy, with its wish for or resentment of manhood, is not a primary difficulty but rather a defensive system against the greater difficulty of being a woman.

CHAPTER 10

The Need to Control

The Nature of Frigidity

The world's literature – fiction and nonfiction – abounds with descriptions and classifications of frigid womanhood. Many serious workers have produced studies both of the statistical estimations of the size of the problem, and of the personality types concerned.

Studies of the treatment of frigidity are less common. The purpose of this book is not to add to the list of psychological classifications by putting our own labels upon the various types of case we encounter, but rather to indicate in outline a technique of treatment we have found effective with a large number of individual, unique, troubled human beings. As a senior colleague aptly said, 'We don't have cases of, we have people who.'

In this final chapter, therefore, I wish to refer only briefly to the view we have acquired of the nature of frigidity through our clinical experience, drawing the reader's attention yet again to the way in which the awareness of the feeling between ourselves and each patient is at every moment our most effective diagnostic tool, and stressing yet again how this and the presenting symptoms often provide the essential determinant of our focus of therapy.

Briefly, we have come to see frigidity as a defensive system against the unconscious fear of the total exposure of the deepest self, which abandonment to vaginal orgasm within the act of intercourse demands. The defensive system, unique and specific to each individual, is acquired and built up through the growing-up process by all of us in varying degrees, in relation to what may be called the 'civilizing' factors in our upbringing. As we mature as members first of a family, later of a wider society, we develop controls over the primitive impulses that childhood implies but adult society finds untidy and unacceptable. These untidy, vulnerable aspects of babyishness are many-sided, and different aspects are more important than others for different people. When the control grows in a secure, loving setting and becomes wholly conscious, the result is a mature and an emotionally free adult, capable of relating fully and confidently to others. When, however, the process is disturbed by early relational difficulties, these primitive needs become associated with anxiety. The individual 'controls' them, in defence against the dangers they imply, by relegating them to the unconscious. The fear develops that to show oneself totally is to show something unlovable, vulnerable, dirty – whatever primitive uncontrolled, undefended babyishness has come to mean to that individual. This process affects, of course, all facets of development, many of which will be the concern of the psychiatrist.

Sexual intercourse is, however, one way in which a patient is brought face to face with such difficulties. As has been stressed repeatedly, vaginal orgasm within the act of intercourse requires a total abandonment of civilized veneers and defences; a total exposure, and sharing with another, of the deepest, most primitive layers of the emotional self. It is simply not compatible with 'Sunday-best' behaviour. The seminar has often found that a patient indeed needs to become 'as a little child' before she can dare to enter this part of the kingdom of heaven.

It is hoped that, from the detailed case studies with which I end the book, the reader will gain two important indications of the special features of this work.

First, this is an empirical technique in which the doctor–patient relationship provides the key at any given moment. The patient is showing us her defensive system – the face she has come unconsciously to need to present to the world. If we can, through our own insight into our reactions to her, recognize the nature of that defensive system, we shall receive a clue to the nature of her fears – of what she needs to hide. Interpretation of the defensive system as she shows it to us in the here-and-now interview, will allow her to look at a part of herself she is hiding – from herself as well as from the world and from us. If we can then accept it and pay tribute to it, she will herself become able to accept it as no longer shameful or frightening, but as a rich talent to be shared in the total commitment that is human sexual love.

Second, I hope these accounts will demonstrate that we regard our task with our patient not as a clinical exercise of examination, appraisal, diagnosis, and classification, followed by magical therapeutic action when possible; but rather as a living relationship in which, and through which, a woman is enabled to allow herself to grow.

Case Studies

Mrs A illustrates how a simple observation of the effect she had on the doctor was more useful than prolonged technical consultation – either physical or psychological – without insight.

She was awaiting surgery for five years' nonconsummation, and crept into the clinic like a frightened mouse, wearing no make-up and speaking almost inaudibly. Every attempt at intercourse from the first night until now had made her scream and scream. She just could not help it. The doctor's heart sank, and on the couch the patient

61

cowered away at once, whispering 'no, no'. Over a period of two months the doctor soothed and cajoled as with a frightened child, until full vaginal examination was possible and the patient could examine herself obediently. The seminar pointed out to the doctor how she was protectively mothering this girl without understanding or interpreting how the patient made her do so. Spurred thus on, the doctor undertook several further sessions, now of psychological exploration. These revealed a previous nervous break-down, and various exciting fantasies in which the patient was victim of frightening – exciting – attacks; all very interesting, but no progress towards intercourse was made.

Then one day the husband waylaid the doctor in deep distress because his wife had left him. They had quarrelled, he had hit her in exasperation, and was now abject in remorse. Suddenly the doctor saw the patient, not as a helpless child, but as a powerful woman controlling husband and doctor alike. She faced the patient with this at the next interview, and the patient was able to accept with surprise that she had this hidden savage side to herself. The marriage was consummated that night, and Mrs A could hardly wait to bring the doctor the news.

Mrs B seemed to be suffering bravely. She was plump, thirty, slovenly in appearance, and wanted a cap because the sheath 'hurt so'. The dyspareunia persisted for days and before it was gone her husband wanted 'it' again. She had had several repairs since her first baby in an attempt to cure this, but all had failed. She used to have clitoral orgasm, but now refused it because she felt it prevented her achieving 'the real thing'. The doctor felt this insistence on physical causes must be a denial of feeling, and expressed doubt that she had ever really enjoyed intercourse. The patient tearfully agreed and began to present herself as the victim of her husband's excessive demands, saying through her tears, 'Take no notice, doctor, I am always like this when I talk of such things.' With the doctor's encouraging attitude, she made some progress with the cap and was able to say she now felt clitoral orgasm was all right; but the improvement was brief. She returned demanding the pill and saying her husband's demands were terrible – he wanted 'it' so often that she became sore and she only need brush past him for him to become aroused.

The doctor suggested she could only see herself as the victim of an unfeeling brute, rather than the fortunate wife of a loving and passionate man.

This girl was warm and at ease in the maternal role when her children came to the clinic and the doctor discussed her attitude to womanhood. She had always been a tomboy, preferring horses to dolls, and both admiring and envying her athletic brother. She felt man had the best of the bargain and did not value being a woman and having a vagina. The doctor was now able to put her in touch with the lively excitement underlying all this. The patient then left the district. Another seminar doctor met her later and found her groomed and feminine in appearance, speaking of her husband's demands with a shy pride, saying that she could use the cap and that everything was now 'perfectly all right'.

Mrs C was virtuous.

Married two years, at twenty-four, her dress was more suited to a Victorian dowager and she fingered a silver cross at her bosom. She had no wish for intercourse, but had agreed to come for treatment of non-consummation because 'It was God's will that it was necessary to marriage'. She was quite passive over examination but revealed such distaste over examining her own vagina that the doctor found herself blushing and feeling she had made a most improper suggestion. On receiving an interpretation, however, the patient claimed ignorance, and was resentful of the doctor refusing to give her information and hints. It

63

was all right, she said, for other people who knew these things. The doctor interpreted her need for ignorance and to be told – it was wicked to know. The patient could now be shown where to put her fingers, and learned to stretch herself and to use a cap obediently like a child.

After this depressing interview, the patient arrived looking so young and gay that the doctor did not recognize her. Examination was quite easy, and she had used the cap correctly. She again claimed, however, that she did not know as much as other people, and there was an angry exchange about how they – and the doctor – kept things from her. She needed to be told. This interpretation enabled her to confess that she feared things would go through from the vagina into the rectum. This, and the associated idea of nastiness, was related by the doctor to her fears of intercourse – that it would be both painful and nasty, and that ideas about it were both damaging and evil.

At the third visit Mrs C was lively and blooming, saying that penetration was 'almost complete'. She was very happy that at last 'she knew what she wanted', but she felt that they now had to do it 'for themselves'. We have found that this new-found independence from the doctor is often the confirmatory sign that the patients can now own their own desires.

Mrs D fainted at cap-fitting.

Coming premaritally at the age of thirty, this competent and businesslike nursery teacher then insisted upon the pill. She said that she had also fainted on trying to use Tampax. At this first visit, the doctor and nurse, not specially trained, were unable to pay tribute to the importance of this unspoken communication of anxiety. At the second visit, to the seminar doctor, she controlled the interview by her 'I know as much about it as you do' attitude. At examination she insisted that she knew all about voluntary muscle relaxation. The doctor remarked that she treated the whole matter very sensibly and clinically and could express no unruly feelings – yet she evidently had needed to faint the first time.

The patient was then able to talk about her chosen husband, younger than she, and how she controlled him by making all the decisions. She had made him shave his moustache, but was disappointed at the less manly result. The doctor observed that she had made him less of a man, and the doctor less of a doctor, by treating them as she treated her young charges. However, in the husband's case the result seemed to sadden her. Mrs D admitted that part of her regretted her controlling tendencies and wished to be more feminine and weak. Gradually she began to see how powerful was her need to control others, and she admitted that she longed for a baby, but felt that she could not manage one yet. This was related by the doctor to the baby – the weak, dependent person – inside herself, which seemed so vulnerable.

After some four months Mrs D could achieve regular orgasm even with the cap, to which she had changed as 'the pill seemed too sure'. She was speaking with pride of her husband's promotion at work – and in the marital relationship also.

Mrs E was angry.

She originally complained of disliking intercourse because of pain, and at examination produced severe adductor spasms of the thighs, which we often find suggests an angry, fighting mood in contrast with the vaginismus of fear. She thought she was too small, and then that there was a wall inside. Encouraged to go on talking, she said she thought the penis would have to go right through the cervical os and that this would be very painful. She also said that if she could allow full penetration (*sic*, into her feelings) that her whole life would be torn up by the roots.

F

Next time she was encouraged to examine herself. She again produced fantasies of being damaged, saying that her husband was inexperienced and might try to go into the urethra.

This critical communication led to discussion of her contemptuous feelings towards men. She said the best thing about being a woman was to make men crawl. She liked to think she could twist them round her little finger. She spoke disparagingly, however, about those women who stayed at home playing bridge or looking after house and children.

Later, Mrs E could discuss her early relationships. She had a belligerent relationship with her father, whom she provoked into anger and glorified in defeating. She always referred to the childhood home as her mother's house, and still went every day to see her mother and to have her dinner. Mother had discovered her sexual difficulties and it was she who had taken her to the doctor. The patient said it made her feel like a small child with measles. Despite the angry feelings about her father, she was at pains to insist that he 'did not count'. Once after a row with her husband she had run home to mother. Although she soon felt able to return to him, her mother had sat up all night crying and begging her to stay.

This patient began to show the change in her feelings about her mother in the way she treated the doctor – coming regularly but making her feel useless.

She agreed she was angry with her mother for allowing her to grow up 'without knowing anything', and wished she would not do so much for her, yet she found herself continuing to seek her mother's help for things she knew she should do for herself. After one angry interview, Mrs E and the doctor mutually agreed to suspend treatment.

On her voluntary return, Mrs E spoke of her dog. He had been very much hers but was now only interested in her husband. The doctor suggested she felt herself her mother's baby, who had now turned her attentions towards her father. She replied, 'I am sure my father wanted to do things for me – but mother would have said he was no good at it.' The patient and doctor then discussed together her difficulty in seeing her father – indeed any man – as both competent and loving, so that she could trust herself to him. She was now able to show the tender dependent part of herself which she had always hidden behind belligerent defensiveness.

The next week she returned saying proudly that they had had intercourse and it was marvellous. Asked how she thought this had happened, she said in her old destructive fashion, 'I suppose it was the thought of having to keep coming to see you!' But the next day a letter of thanks arrived with a beautiful bunch of flowers.

Mrs F was an efficient businesswoman.

A newly married, very 'with-it' young Canadian came with her husband, who worked with her in a big advertising agency, asking for the pill. They thought it might help her to achieve orgasm, which was always just out of reach with the sheath. She had prevailed upon her husband to bring her, but was sure that she herself was at fault.

The first interview was businesslike, with the doctor insisting that the pill itself was unlikely to help and that they would have to go into her feelings. The moment of truth at first examination was a negative one. She tolerated examination without revealing any feelings and fitted her cap in the same competent way. This, then, was the truth. Her outer defence was brisk efficiency.

At the next session, to which she came alone, she was sullen and demanded answers to practical questions about the technique of intercourse. The doctor found this abusive attitude a strain, but noted and used it rather than answering the questions. 'I can see you are irritated with me for not giving you a magical answer. It is hard for you to admit that you need help, yet you seem to expect other people to do it

67

all for you.' This was an angry struggling interview with no facts emerging except her resentment at her need to depend on other people for help. It was pointed out in the seminar that in a sense she had controlled this interview too by making a fight of it.

However, next time she talked in a natural and dependent way. Several layers of cosmetics had also been shed. She went so far as to say, 'I know my only hope is coming to talk to you.' On examination she was very different. She was shy, blushing, and relaxed. The doctor said during the examination, 'You seem to feel differently about it this time?' 'Well, I know it is silly, but I am afraid I have cancer or something nasty inside.' This was interpreted, 'I can tell you there's no growth, but it seems to me your feelings about your inside have something to do with it. Perhaps you feel there is something nasty about them?'

Sitting down, the patient revealed that she would like to have her husband take charge, go back to the sheath, and really 'make' her. The doctor said, 'Yes, you really have some quite exciting ideas about how it should be. But it is difficult for the sensible side of you to let him, or to let your own feelings go.' The patient joked that she would tell him, 'The doctor says you must drag me around by the hair.' The doctor replied that she did not mind taking the blame for now but, when the patient could ask it for herself, that would really be progress! A last-minute communication in the waiting-room when no further talk was possible was, 'What I would really like is a baby.'

Seminar discussion suggested it was the baby side of herself with which she needed to be put in touch, and there was some general speculation whether she might be an only child or the eldest of the family. Dr Main discouraged this as being theorizing not based on the evidence at hand. He was proved right when the next visit demonstrated the futility of trying to substantiate preconceived ideas.

The husband had received the (allegedly doctor's)

suggestion about getting tough with, 'It's all right for her –
you'd only slap me down.' This, like all quotes from other
people, was interpreted as something the patient felt herself.
Intercourse had been better since the last visit, interestingly
after a quarrel, paralleling the improved response after her
fighting interview with the doctor. She had then been ill
and had to 'just lie around', her husband having to do
everything around the house. This delightfully symbolic
communication was interpreted and led to further discussion of who had to be in charge. The patient said that she
could now make advances, but at the last minute 'nothing,
a waste of time'. This was related to the way she treated the
doctor, with lots of exciting talk, but when they seemed to
be getting somewhere she pulled back and slapped the
doctor down, saying that it was all a waste of time.

The doctor, under tension after this heated exchange,
conveniently remembered her last-minute communication
at the previous consultation and the seminar discussion!
'About this wanting a baby?' *Patient*: 'Yes, it seems silly to
be taking precautions.' *Doctor*: 'Are you an only child?'
Patient (blankly): 'No, one of three.' *Doctor*: 'The eldest,
perhaps?' *Patient* (blanker still!): 'No, the second!'

The doctor then realized what was happening, collected
her wits, and tried again with an interpretation of the
patient's attitude. 'I was thinking when you talked of wanting a baby, how difficult it is for you to be a baby yourself.'
This did produce something. 'Well, I was the only one sent
away to school. I was only twelve. I know Mom did it for
the best, but I guess I was too young really to stand on my
own two feet.' Talk about her feelings at this time revealed
that there was no place for tears and foolishness at school,
and that she missed Mom most. Father, though not discussed much, was 'very close, always good for a bit of fun
and rough and tumble', while Mom and school were clearly
on the side of law and order.

Interpretation of this feeling of being too young led to

69

discussion of the feeling that she was herself too young to be married. She examined herself with feeling now for the first time. She was blushing and pleased, surprised that her vagina was bigger and nicer than she had thought. There was more talk of how things were easier for her when she was bullied into them. She then confided that she would like to give up her job and spend more time on the house, but feared that if she did so she would have time on her hands to sit around thinking silly feminine thoughts. This conflict within herself was again interpreted – the silly, babyish, adventurous, but dependent side with feminine wishes, versus the defensive, independent grown-up career girl.

At the last visit she had given up her job for part-time freelancing, so that she could choose her hours and spend more time on the house (*sic*). She had had orgasm once or twice, and her husband was thrilled. She said she had changed completely in herself and that all her friends were commenting on her improved appearance. When they said that marriage suited her, she and her husband would look at each other and laugh!

The patient did not keep her next appointment and it was a year later when the doctor found her walking past her house, which was some way from the main road, pushing a lovely baby girl in a beautifully decorated pram. The patient said she was only passing by, but the doctor was thrilled to be allowed to see this evidence of her femininity.

Mrs G was at odds with her domestic role.

Presently with an urgent marital difficulty after seven years, she appeared and acted like an attractive teenager, in jeans and casual hairstyle. The doctor was surprised to hear that she was twenty-six and the mother of two children. She burst out at once with a torrent of superfluous information, saying the marriage was on the rocks as she had never had an orgasm. She found great difficulty in coping with the chores and her two boys were too much for her. Her husband, a writer, stayed working in the attic, and she felt shut out, useless, and ignorant. The doctor interpreted her resentment and heard how her own education had been paltry. Her mother was talented and lovely and 'could have done anything' but was content for the whole household to be directed and bullied by an erratic father.

The doctor allowed her to air her resentments and showed to her her contempt for her mother and for woman's role in the family. She agreed with emotion and also expressed her anger at her father's domination. Encouraged to pursue this high feeling, Mrs G disclosed a sense of deep humiliation at her father's repeated incestuous advances to her, hitherto undisclosed to anyone. She was very shaken at having revealed so much and the doctor sensed both anger and anxiety as she left saying, 'How is all this talking going to help?'

Next time the patient tried to re-establish control of the interview and the doctor interpreted her need to control both her anger and her anxieties. Now the shadowy figure of her husband in his ivory tower began to take shape, and she discussed her resentment of him and related it to her feelings about her father. She was particularly afraid of the humiliation of submitting to him and thus conceding the control she had fostered. Now she could see with delight how her feelings were operating, and could admit that many of her difficulties with husband and children were of her own making. She would provoke the situations that she then resented.

One month later Mrs G was self-possessed and wearing an elegant dress. She said she was enjoying intercourse though she did not always achieve orgasm. She asked to be fitted with a cap for the first time in four years, and agreed that she was more at ease with her femininity. She rather enjoyed the household chores now, and the boys were less trouble because she handled them better. She realized that

71

being intellectually inferior to her husband and friends did not matter, and she had arranged a warm room for her husband to work in downstairs. 'Like a warm vagina?' suggested the doctor – Mrs G was delighted to have worked it out for herself.

Mrs H thought she had a cloaca.

A girl of twenty-three, she was already a university graduate in zoology and had just started in a teaching post of some distinction, when she came pre-maritally for a cap. She was sensible and businesslike. When examined, the hymen admitted only one finger. The doctor, not specially trained in marital difficulties, could only reassure her and suggest using Tampax. She was asked to come back in a week.

Next time she had been unable to insert the Tampax, and again this complaint of physical disability was taken at its face value by the doctor, who considered that it would be impossible to fit her with a cap before her marriage. She asked her to practise digital stretching and to return after the wedding. It is impossible to blame either the patient or the doctor for this. The doctor was unable to interpret the underlying anxiety because her classical training equipped her only to ask factual questions admitting of straight answers, and to assess physical problems as physical entities. The patient was unable to reveal her anxiety because her whole outer personality was one of independent good sense; the more so because she had unconscious fears to hide.

In the event, despite the warm reassurance and encouragement she had received, it took her nine months to find the courage to come again, during which time the marriage had not been consummated. Next time she met one of the seminar doctors.

She admitted now that the cap-check was a flimsy pretext for her visit, and that the marriage had not been consummated. On examination, the hymen still admitted only one finger, and her attitude was of a pupil seeking instruction. This doctor did not accept this physical problem at its face value, but instead remarked that examination seemed to be a great ordeal for her. She showed her how to contract and relax her perineal muscles and encouraged her to put her own finger in to explore the vagina. This caused reluctance and nausea, which were discussed, and eventually a cap was fitted and taken away for practice.

Two weeks later she returned to say she had been unable to remove the cap and needed further help to do so. The doctor persisted in trying to discuss her feelings about her genitals, but the patient was unable to put her fears into words. Next time she had managed the cap and there was a marked decrease in vaginismus, but she now said that intercourse was impossible because her husband could no longer get an erection. There was a long discussion of his sexual inadequacy, with the patient denying her own part in the problem entirely. An appointment was made for him to see a psychiatrist, who gave a gloomy prognosis. For a further three visits the situation remained the same and the husband no longer attempted intercourse.

Seminar discussion suggested that the patient must somehow be helped to see her own part in the problem. At the next visit the vaginismus had returned and the patient's bluff was called. It was put to her that she could not admit that she herself had any emotional difficulty. Now the atmosphere between the doctor and patient became more honest and warm and the patient admitted, 'You know, the trouble was really that I thought there was only one opening.' The doctor accepted this fantasy without ridicule, and allowed the patient to go on to elaborate that she felt she had a cloaca like the animals she had learned about in biology. She talked freely about childhood difficulties with her genital area, when she had suffered from chronic frequency and urgency of micturition for many years. She had

73

become so terrified of catheterization that she had to have an anaesthetic. She felt that she had only this one small opening, and that intercourse would be terribly painful and damaging.

Immediately after this interview, consummation took place, the husband's potency miraculously restored! She returned saying that life was quite different now and that they were not bothering to use the cap because they hoped to start a baby.

We have tried honestly to show that not all our cases go as well as this and that we as doctors are still far from perfect in the technique we have developed. Nor does every doctor who enters training find either the aptitude or indeed the taste for working at this level.

We suspect also that the technique in itself has far to go, and may in years to come have far wider application than we can give it today.

The transformation in successful cases, however, seems to have such impact on the patient's whole personality and capacity for living and loving, that had we had only one success of the many described, we should regard our five years of experience as well spent.

Index

abandonment, 10, 60
abnormality, fears of, 8, 9
abortion, effects of, 9, 22, 52, 53
adoption, effects of, 29, 30
aggressive behaviour, 4, 35
aggressive feelings, 3
anxiety
    exploration of, 13
    on exploration of genitals, 11.
       See also, vaginal examina-
       tion
    non-verbalized, 23
    of premarital patients, 44
    about showing weakness or
       dependency, 3
    about vagina, *see under*
       vagina
    virginal, 43–8
'athletic' approach to sexual
    act, 2

babyishness, 16, 30, 60, 70
baby, longing for, 29, 65, 68, 69
Balint, Michael, xi, xiv, 43
behaviour
    aggressive, 4, 35
    civilized, 8
    communications by, 20
    'Sunday-best', 10, 60
birth-control, *see* contraceptive
    methods
'blanket' approach to patients,
    1

brief-encounter therapy, 3
'Brunhild' concept, 43, 56

cancer, fear of, 10, 25, 28, 68
cap
    difficulties, 40
    enjoyment of intercourse
       with, 37
    loss of orgasm with, 37
    pregnancy with, 40
cap-fitting
    anxiety at, 23
    difficulty in, 22
    moment of truth at, 7
cap-teaching, 7, 9, 10–11
case histories, *see under* patient
childbirth, frigidity after, 50–3
childhood experiences, effects
    of, 37, 47, 69
clinic, *see under* Family Plan-
    ning Association
clitoral orgasm, *see under* org-
    asm
coitus interruptus, 29, 31, 38
collusion, with patient, 28, 32
combined pill, *see under* pill
communication,
    last-minute, 24–6, 68, 69
    unspoken, 20–6
conception
    as purpose of intercourse,
       see under sexual inter-
       course